'This book is a breath of fresh air that blows through dusty institutionalised psychoanalytic corridors, cleansing them of sectarian dogma and theoretical driftwood. This collection of essays is independent thinking at its best; it is a real eye (and heart) opener. It might be a cliché, but it is true nevertheless: it needs to be read by every supervisor, and more importantly, by every psychoanalytic training institution.'

Farhad Dalal, *Psychotherapist and Group Analyst, UK;*
Director of Training, Group Analysis, India, Bengaluru

'Working therapeutically can at times be daunting for even the most experienced practitioners when we are faced with unthinkable trauma and psychic pain experienced by the children and families we work with. Yet good supervision makes it possible. Here some of the most respected child psychotherapists of their time with decades of clinical experience, show how supervision can be transformational in guiding practitioners in their work, helping to hold and think about difficulty whilst enabling them to find their own voice in their therapeutic practice. This assembly of carefully curated wisdom is a much needed addition to our reading and thinking.'

Jane O'Rourke, *Psychodynamic Child, Adolescent and*
Family Psychotherapist, and Founder of MINDinMIND

'This very welcome volume from the independent psychoanalytic child and adolescent psychotherapy tradition is long overdue. It covers different aspects of clinical supervision in a variety of settings and brings many of the tensions that supervisors, practitioners and trainees grapple with, in an engaging way. The supervisory superego is one that is inevitably ubiquitous but the papers in this collection address the contradictory task faced in the supervisory process, of transmission of the psychoanalytic tradition at the same time as facilitating the clinician to use their own creativity in their learning and development. It is to be recommended to supervisors and trainees alike.'

Angela Joyce, *Fellow of the BPAS; Training and Supervising*
Psychoanalyst of Adults and Children

Supervision in a Changing World

Supervision in a Changing World explores the range of skills and knowledge a child and adolescent psychotherapist brings to the practice of supervision.

Featuring contributions from leading child psychotherapists drawing on their clinical and supervisory experiences, chapters highlight a range of individual supervision approaches. Key issues covered include the history of thinking around supervision; ethical considerations; the interplay between the supervisee and supervisor experience; the complexities of service supervision; working with trauma; and supervising work with children and adolescents with disabilities. The book will also give direct insight into preparing process notes and report writing, research supervision, supervising colleagues in different settings and countries and the training school perspective. Attention is also paid to diversity and power dynamics and the implications of 'remote' supervision (both before and since Covid-19).

One of the few works specifically dedicated to child psychoanalytic psychotherapy supervision, this book aims to meet the needs of child psychotherapist supervisors and those training to become supervisors. It will also be useful for professionals in allied professions, and those who are interested in therapeutic work with children.

Deirdre Dowling is a child, adolescent and adult psychoanalytic psychotherapist in private practice in Surrey, UK. She is also a teacher and supervisor. Previously, she worked on the Family Service at the Cassel Hospital, an NHS residential therapeutic assessment and treatment service, and at the British Foundation for Psychotherapy (bpf) as Curriculum Lead for the Independent Child and Adolescent Psychoanalytic Psychotherapy Association (IPCAPA) training.

Julie Kitchener is a teacher and training supervisor for IPCAPA at the bpf. Currently in independent practice, she has worked as a child and adolescent psychotherapist in both general and specialist NHS Child and Adolescent Mental Health Services, and for many years was lead psychotherapist in a children's residential community.

Independent Psychoanalytic Approaches with Children and Adolescents series
Series Editors: Ann Horne and Teresa Bailey

Supervision in a Changing World

Reflections from Child Psychotherapy

Edited by Deirdre Dowling and Julie Kitchener

Routledge
Taylor & Francis Group

LONDON AND NEW YORK

Designed cover image: © Photodisc & ImageDJ / Design Master

First published 2024
by Routledge
4 Park Square, Milton Park, Abingdon, Oxon OX14 4RN

and by Routledge
605 Third Avenue, New York, NY 10158

Routledge is an imprint of the Taylor & Francis Group, an informa business

© 2024 selection and editorial matter, Deirdre Dowling and Julie Kitchener; individual chapters, the contributors

British Library Cataloguing-in-Publication Data
A catalogue record for this book is available from the British Library

Library of Congress Cataloging-in-Publication Data
Names: Dowling, Deirdre, editor. | Kitchener, Julie, editor.
Title: Supervision in a changing world : reflections from child psychotherapy / edited by Deirdre Dowling and Julie Kitchener.
Description: Abingdon, Oxon ; New York, NY : Routledge, 2024. |
Series: Independent psychoanalytic approaches with children and adolescents |
Includes bibliographical references and index.
Identifiers: LCCN 2023010989 (print) | LCCN 2023010990 (ebook) |
ISBN 9781032285979 (hardback) | ISBN 9781032286006 (paperback) |
ISBN 9781003297604 (ebook)
Subjects: LCSH: Child psychotherapists–Supervision of. |
Child psychotherapists–Training of. |
Child psychotherapy–Study and teaching.
Classification: LCC RJ504 .S834 2024 (print) |
LCC RJ504 (ebook) | DDC 618.92/8914–dc23/eng/20230607
LC record available at https://lccn.loc.gov/2023010989
LC ebook record available at https://lccn.loc.gov/2023010990

ISBN: 9781032285979 (hbk)
ISBN: 9781032286006 (pbk)
ISBN: 9781003297604 (ebk)

DOI: 10.4324/9781003297604

Typeset in Times New Roman
by Newgen Publishing UK

In memory of Mani Vastardis, a beloved supervisor, colleague and friend

Contents

Contributors

Evrinomy Avdi is an associate professor of clinical psychology at the Aristotle University of Thessaloniki, Greece, and research tutor in the Doctorate in Child and Adolescent Psychotherapy at the Independent Psychoanalytic Child and Adolescent Psychotherapy Association at the British Psychotherapy Foundation (IPCAPA at the bpf)/ University College London. She is director of the Laboratory of Applied Psychology at the School of Psychology, Aristotle University, which provides psychotherapy services to the community, as well as training and supervision to mental health professionals, and she conducts research. She has trained in dramatherapy, clinical psychology and adult psychoanalytic psychotherapy; she teaches undergraduate and postgraduate courses in psychology and supervises clinical psychologists and psychotherapists in their clinical work and in research. Her research interests lie in using qualitative methods – particularly discursive and narrative research – to study the process of psychotherapy, as well as the experience of serious illness.

Teresa Bailey was Head of Psychoanalytic Psychotherapy for Oxleas Foundation Trust before she retired from the National Health Service (NHS). She devised and ran IPCAPA intensive case supervisors' training courses for experienced child psychotherapists. In Oxleas, she trained senior Band 7 and Band 8 child psychotherapists to supervise the clinical work of colleagues and trainees. She continues to offer clinical and management consultation to a range of mental health professionals including to senior child psychotherapists. One day a week, she volunteers at the Baobab Centre for young survivors/asylum seekers. She has an MA in screen writing and writes mostly female-led drama.

Pamela Bartram is a child, adolescent and adult psychoanalytic psychotherapist working in private practice. She has roles in assessing, teaching and supervising at the British Foundation for Psychotherapy (bpf). She chairs the bpf Infant Observation Committee and teaches infant observation for clinical trainees and external students. She started her career as a music therapist where much of her work was with children with disabilities. After training as a child and adolescent psychotherapist, she became a clinician/manager in the NHS and contributed to the design and delivery of a multi-agency service for children with disabilities and their families. She has a special interest in the mutative effect in the clinical encounter of the nonverbal aspects of human communication, especially play and unconscious communication.

Diana Cant is a consultant child psychotherapist, living and working in Kent, who originally trained at the Tavistock Clinic. Although no longer doing direct work, she still offers supervision and consultation. Much of her professional life has been spent working in therapeutic communities, including the Henderson Hospital, the Caldecott Community and Childhood First, and accounts of this work have been published in the *Journal of Child Psychotherapy*. Recently she has returned to writing poetry and her pamphlet, *At Risk – The Lives Some Children Live* (2021), reflects both of her interests. She was poet in residence for the Association of Child Psychotherapists (ACP) Conference, 2021, and nominated for the Forward prize for best individual poem, 2023.

Francine Conway is an award-winning child psychologist and Chancellor-Provost of Rutgers University, New Brunswick. Formerly Dean of the Graduate School of Applied Professional Psychology at Rutgers, she is also a highly experienced clinician, treating children in hospital settings and private practice for more than 20 years. She has gained national and international recognition for her achievements in the fields of attention deficit hyperactivity disorder (ADHD) and black mental health and diversity, as well as her commitment to driving social change. Her particular interest in disability and learning difficulties has led Dr Conway to integrate services and research programmes for the support needs and life-span of people with autism at Rutgers. She is the founder and director of the 'Cultivating Compassion ADHD Project', a funded clinical specialty training programme providing psychodynamic training and treatment for children with ADHD, and has an ongoing research project 'Cultivating Compassion: Mentalization-Based Treatment for ADHD'. Dr Conway also serves as the research editor for the *Journal of Infant, Child and Adolescent Psychotherapy.* Her latest book is *Cultivating Compassion: A Psychodynamic Understanding of Attention Deficit Hyperactivity Disorder.*

Martin Daltrop is a consultant child and adolescent psychotherapist in a South London NHS Trust, having qualified in 2003 from the British Association of Psychotherapists (now IPCAPA at the bpf). Since qualification, he has worked in various roles in Child and Adolescent Mental Health Services (CAMHS), in several London boroughs, in specialist looked after children (LAC), adoption and adolescent teams as well as in generic CAMHS, treating young people across the age range 0–18. Over the course of the past nine years, he has worked as a service supervisor to qualified clinicians and trainees. In his current role, he is lead child and adolescent psychotherapist, having responsibility for the discipline as a whole within the Trust. He is also part of a leadership group which is responsible for the delivery and planning of the CAMHS within the Trust. He has taught for many years on adult and child trainings and has been an intensive case supervisor.

Deirdre Dowling is a child, adolescent and adult psychoanalytic psychotherapist who trained at the British Psychotherapy Foundation. She is a teacher and supervisor for IPCAPA, where she was the curriculum lead from 2011–2015. Previously, she worked as head child psychotherapist at the Cassel Hospital, an NHS inpatient psychotherapeutic hospital for families in severe difficulties. She has published several chapters and a book entitled *An Independent Practitioner's Introduction to Child and Adolescent Psychotherapy: Playing with Ideas* (2019) in the series Independent Psychoanalytic Approaches with Children and Adolescents published by Routledge. She has a particular interest in consulting to other professionals interested in applying psychoanalytic ideas to their work with children and families and she has taught in multidisciplinary settings both in the UK and overseas.

Iris Gibbs trained as a child and adolescent psychotherapist with the British Association of Psychotherapists (now IPCAPA at the bpf). She is currently a member of staff on the IPCAPA training and teaches, supervises and runs workshops on issues of diversity. She worked for five years at the Anna Freud Centre and was one of the original members of the Parent Infant Project (PIP). She has a private practice and offers supervision to trained therapists and other healthcare professionals. She has also been a consultant to a therapeutic fostering organisation for a number of years and has contributed to the following books: *The Practice of Psychoanalytic Parent-Infant Psychotherapy: Claiming the Baby*, (2005) edited by Tessa Baradon; *A Question of Technique* (2006) and *Through Assessment to Consultation: Independent Psychoanalytic Approaches with Children and Adolescents* (2009), both edited by Monica Lanyado and Ann Horne as part of the Independent Psychoanalytic Approaches with Children and Adolescents series for Routledge.

Ann Horne is a Fellow of the bpf and an Honorary Member of the Czech Society for Psychoanalytic Psychotherapy. Trained as a child psychotherapist at the British Association of Psychotherapists (BAP) (now IPCAPA at the bpf), she was later head of training and then of postgraduate development. A former joint editor of the *Journal of Child Psychotherapy*, she co-edited with Monica Lanyado *The Handbook of Child and Adolescent Psychotherapy: Psychoanalytic Approaches* (1st edition 1999; 2nd edition 2009) and conceived the Independent Psychoanalytic Approaches with Children and Adolescents series for Routledge. Her selected papers (*On Children Who Privilege the Body*) were published by Routledge in 2018. Retired from NHS work, latterly at the Portman Clinic in London, she still retains a particular interest in children who use the body and activity rather than being able to access thought and reflection.

Julie Kitchener is a teacher and training supervisor for IPCAPA at the bpf. She trained as a child and adolescent psychoanalytic psychotherapist at what was then the British Association of Psychotherapy, after following a career in journalism. She has worked in both general and specialist NHS Child and Adolescent Mental Health Services, and for many years was lead psychotherapist then head of therapy in a children's residential therapeutic community. Currently in independent practice, she retains links with local authority and CAMHS, working with children and families as well as consulting to fostering agencies. She previously contributed to *Winnicott's Children* (2012), in the Independent Psychoanalytic Approaches with Children and Adolescents series.

Monica Lanyado is a training supervisor for IPCAPA at the bpf. She was founding course organising tutor of the Child and Adolescent Psychoanalytic Psychotherapy Training at the Scottish Institute of Human Relations (now Human Development Scotland). Now retired from clinical practice, she teaches, lectures and supervises in the UK and internationally. Her publications include *The Presence of the Therapist: Treating Childhood Trauma* (2004) and *Transforming Despair to Hope: Reflections on the Psychotherapeutic Process with Severely Neglected and Traumatised Children* (2018). She has co-edited six books with Ann Horne including *The Handbook of Child and Adolescent Psychotherapy: Psychoanalytic Approaches* (1999, 2009), and four books in the Independent Psychoanalytic Approaches with Children and Adolescents series for which she was joint series editor with Ann Horne from 2005 to 2019. She was joint editor of the *Journal of Child Psychotherapy* from 1995 to 1998.

Coretta Ogbuagu is a principal child and adolescent psychotherapist, leading a psychotherapy team in a CAMHS within the NHS in East London. She has worked in mental health services with babies, older children and adults in a variety of settings for more than a decade. Coretta is also a psychoanalytic parent-infant psychotherapist and provides this specialist treatment in CAMHS. She teaches and supervises on the Sino-British psychoanalytic psychotherapy training programme for children and adolescents in China. Coretta enjoys writing, teaching and giving talks on her clinical experiences at various conferences and events, and on a range of psychoanalytical teaching programmes. She currently supports trainee child and adolescent psychotherapists from the IPCAPA bpf training school as both a service supervisor and progress advisor, giving back to the institution where she trained.

Janine Sternberg was clinical course director until 2022 of the Independent Psychoanalytic Child and Adolescent Psychotherapy training, a University College London accredited clinical doctorate offered jointly by IPCAPA at the bpf and the Anna Freud Centre. Previously she worked as a consultant child psychotherapist at the Portman Clinic, Tavistock and Portman NHS Trust, having worked for many years before that at the Tavistock Mulberry Bush Day Unit, a small unit for children with complex difficulties. She trained originally as a child psychotherapist at the Tavistock Clinic and subsequently as an adult psychotherapist at the British Association of Psychotherapists. She is very involved in training issues and active in the professional body for child psychotherapists, the Association of Child Psychotherapists. She has been editor of the *Journal of Child Psychotherapy* and editorial co-ordinator of the *British Journal of Psychotherapy*. As well as numerous other chapters and briefer publications, she has written a book that addresses what capacities and skills are needed for psychotherapeutic work and how these may be enhanced by infant observation, *Infant Observation at the Heart of Training* (2005) and co-edited, with Cathy Urwin, a book on infant observation as a research methodology, *Infant Observation and Research: Emotional Processes in Everyday Lives* (2012), both published by Routledge.

Lydia Tischler is a Fellow of the British Psychotherapy Foundation (bpf) and currently a teaching member of the staff at IPCAPA. She is a graduate of the Hampstead Child Therapy training, graduating in 1957. Lydia joined the British Association of Psychotherapy (now bpf) in 1984 and was chair of the Child and Adolescent Training Committee, 1991–1994 and 2001–2005, and chair of Council, 1995–1998. Between 1991 and 2003, Lydia held various positions within the Association of Child Psychotherapists, of which she is an Honoured Member, including chair of the Training Council, 2001–2004. She was a founder member of the European Federation of Psychoanalytic Psychotherapy (EFPP), initiated the training programme in child and adolescent psychotherapy in the Czech Republic in 1995 and, over the years, taught in Estonia, St Petersburg and in Croatia at the Psychoanalytic Institute for Eastern Europe summer school for child and adolescent psychoanalysis. Lydia has published a number of articles on her work at the Cassel Hospital and co-edited *The Family as Inpatient* (1987). Her article 'Anna Freud: A new look at development' was published in the *British Journal of Psychotherapy* in 2014.

Ben Yeo is a child and adolescent psychoanalytic psychotherapist who trained at IPCAPA. Ben currently works in independent practice and with families and children aged pre-birth to four in a Parent and Infant Relationship Service in CAMHS. Prior to training, Ben worked as a family engagement manager in East London and for the Children's Commissioner for England. He is also National Clinical Advisor at the Parent Infant Foundation. Ben won the Louise Emanuel Essay Prize for Infant Mental Health in 2019.

Acknowledgements

We are indebted to Ann Horne and Monica Lanyado for recognising the importance of gathering the ideas that inform and inspire child psychotherapists working
in the Independent psychoanalytic tradition, and who brought those ideas to life
in this series. Thanks, too, to Teresa Bailey for continuing the tradition alongside
Ann. It was Ann who identified the need for a book on supervision written by child
and adolescent psychotherapists, and *Supervision in a Changing World* was her
conception. We are delighted to have had the opportunity to see the project through
and to have been given the freedom to do so in our own way. Nonetheless, our work
as editors would not have been possible without Ann's tactful oversight and eagle-
eyed proof-reading. Our husbands, Harry and Damian also deserve a mention for
their patience, presence and support.

A particular thank you to Diana Cant for her lyrical encapsulation of the supervisory experience, 'Flight path' – a poem she wrote especially for this book.

We are grateful to Taylor & Francis Ltd and the editors of the *Journal of Child
Psychotherapy* for permission to use M Lanyado's (2016) 'Transforming despair to hope in the treatment of extreme trauma: a view from the supervisor's
chair' *Journal of Child Psychotherapy* 42(2): 107–121. Chapter 2 is a version of
a paper presented at the Anna Freud National Centre for Children and Families
Colloquium in November 2021. Thanks to participants for their comments and
reflections.

This is a book that draws, first and foremost, on the experience of supervision.
It is, therefore, the culmination of many diverse supervisory encounters and discussions. We are grateful to all those whose contributions to each of the various
writers are acknowledged in their chapters – peer group, co-trainees, supervisees
and supervisors and those who have taught in this country and abroad. In a book
about supervision, writers are mindful of complex issues of confidentiality –
bearing a responsibility to patients, families, supervisees, supervisors and colleagues. This means that, even where permissions have been sought and granted,
details have necessarily been disguised or changed, and illustrative vignettes
imaginatively re-created from the experience of working with a variety of

individuals who may also share common themes. It is not possible to name each of these 'invisible' contributors, but the authors owe significant thanks to all their supervisors and supervisees past and present for the ideas and insights they have shared. And, finally, thank you to the children whose development has been enabled by those who recognise the necessity to seek supervision.

Foreword

Francine Conway, Rutgers University,
New Brunswick, USA

The book *Supervision in a Changing World: Reflections from Child Psychotherapy* addresses a void in child psychotherapy by offering a rich and thoughtful discourse on the complex and multifaceted issue of child psychotherapy supervision. I approached this book through a lens informed by my experiences as a clinical psychologist, doctoral faculty and researcher. My perspective is also informed by my experience in providing psychodynamic therapy for traumatised children and young people diagnosed with attention deficit hyperactivity disorder (ADHD). From this perspective, I appreciate the critical and timely questions the book raises about the role of supervision for any professional working with vulnerable groups.

'Supervisors oversee the work of others' (*Webster's Dictionary*). The supervisor and supervisee's relationship is the cornerstone of psychotherapy among psychotherapists. Supervisors establish the parameters for the relationship. For example, supervisors ensure confidentiality; adopt a listening stance; encourage curiosity and creativity; and support the reflections of the supervisee. Equally important, supervisors work to create an environment where the supervisee can deepen their understanding and appreciate the complexities of the work. However, child psychotherapy supervision extends beyond other types of supervision in some critical ways. It occurs in a complex multidimensional matrix of interwoven elements. *Supervision in a Changing World* discusses the perspectives of the supervisor and supervisee in diverse settings and against current cultural and societal challenges. Together, the chapters present the *dimensions of child psychotherapy supervision* as a dialectic and invite us all to explore the options, much like the processes in psychodynamic child psychotherapy.

Before considering the dimensions of the supervisor/supervisee's work, I would stress that both therapist and supervisor must acknowledge the complex world of the child – the child's ecosystem. The child's world is composed of a constellation of systems that the child navigates. The individual components of these systems do not necessarily interact or may not even be aware of each other's existence, importance or impact. The most visibly impactful members of this constellation are the parents or caregivers. As children are minors, parents consent to treatment and are responsible for bringing the child to the therapy sessions. The therapist will have to interact with parents, however briefly or extensively, depending on the therapist's therapeutic orientation. Other components of the child's orbit, such as schools/education system and peers, may or may not be accessible to the therapist but constitute a large percentage of the child's world. Less visible contributors include the legal system, which sets standards about how children should be cared for with clearly outlined responsibilities for therapists and other relevant professionals in the network to intervene when these standards are not met. And even less visible are the immediate and extended family interactions and dynamics that may impact the treatment but are not necessarily readily identifiable. These systems shape the child's world, although children have little choice in deciding who inhabits their universe. As a result, the child in psychotherapy treatment is more vulnerable than adult clients, and treatment is hugely dependent on the adults in their lives. Understanding this context is essential for the therapist and the supervisor as they navigate multiple relationship constellations during the treatment.

The dimensions of the supervisor's and supervisee's work are reflected in the poignant stories and case examples underlying their perspectives. While discussing my view of some of the critical dimensions of the supervisory matrix, I believe supervisors' awareness of the inherent dialectic of each dimension is essential. Some of the supervisory matrix dimensions worth elaborating on here include the child's development, the societal challenges stemming from heightened racial and social justice consciousness and the changing therapeutic environment.

One dimension of the supervisory matrix centres on the importance of the child's development. The child's physical and emotional developmental stage is an essential backdrop for evaluating the child's behaviour, especially when the child experiences developmental trauma (see 'Enhancing practice: consultation to a therapeutic fostering agency', Iris Gibbs, Chapter 9). The tension between belonging and the rift trauma visits on one's connection to others requires additional consultation and support for fostering agency teams. Therapists also work with children with other developmental experiences that diverge from what is considered neurotypical. For example, when working with a child with a disability, supervisors can help to guide the therapist to evaluate the disability as part of the 'clinical picture' (see 'Supervising work with children and young people with a disability', Pamela Bartram, Chapter 8). Under these circumstances, Bartram highlights a dimension of supervision that requires balancing the traditional role of the supervisor as offering containment and insight versus providing room for the supervisee to develop their understanding and refine their technique independently. Managing this balance between dependence and independence in supervision will allow the therapist to work through detailed clinical presentations and consider issues of separation and individuation, such as those presented by children with disabilities. In sum, the factors impacting the child's development shape the child's sense of belonging versus feeling isolated or separate, whether it stems from trauma or disability. Simultaneously, the authors highlight the therapist's developmental experience as they balance independence in their thought and technique with dependence on the supervisor.

Another dimension the book addresses is how the heightened public awareness around social justice, spurred by the murder of George Floyd and the Covid pandemic, has shaped the changes psychotherapy has been undergoing. Child therapists have often relied on supervisors for advice on interacting with the child in the therapy session. Especially for newly qualified child therapists, supervisors need to provide guidance on how to be in the 'therapeutic room' with the child. What does the therapist do in the room? How do you sit with a child? How do you play with a child? For example, a child's language development determines whether the treatment will predominantly include imaginative play versus verbal interventions. Issues of diversity and the legacy of the Covid pandemic have significant implications for how these technical issues are addressed in supervision. Working with children requires creativity and the therapist's openness to collaborating with the child in the therapy room as the relationship evolves.

Regarding the social reckoning stemming from the murder of George Floyd, there is increased attention to unconscious biases and privilege in the supervisory relationship and the therapist's relationship with their clients. These social issues raise new questions and contexts for supervision that now must accommodate inquiry (see 'Supervision in extraordinary times', Teresa Bailey, Chapter 7). Supervisors, once viewed as objective and unbiased authorities, are now expected to consider how one's privilege and biases impact the supervisory relationship. At the same time, therapists are forced to grapple with their unconscious biases; they are also faced with managing Covid-19-related changes in the delivery of psychotherapy. The pandemic led to the mandatory isolation of everyone. For the first time in many decades, supervisors, therapists and clients were experiencing the same trauma simultaneously. Supervisors and therapists have had to ensure continuity of service while new professional guidelines were being developed and simultaneously manage their emotional responses.

Moreover, the pandemic has redefined the therapeutic environment from the purely physical therapy room to include the possibility of a virtual one. The therapist must now consider using electronic platforms and other 'remote' technology with the child. In addressing the impact of the pandemic, Bailey highlights the tension between the traditional view of supervisors as all-knowing and the current reality in which supervisors and therapists must discover together this new psychotherapy frontier. Despite the pandemic-related changes, Monica Lanyado ('A view from the supervisor's chair: thoughts on turning points and facilitating hope in therapy through face-to-face and online supervision', Chapter 13) highlights the supervisor's role in balancing the pandemic challenges with finding hope in the face of trauma.

The child's ecosystem and some dimensions of the supervisory matrix – developmental assessment, considerations of societal challenges and the pandemic impact on therapeutic setting and approach – could all be considered external variables in the matrix. But factors intrinsic to the therapist are equally important.

The supervisor must prepare the therapist for the psychological response to working with the child. More specifically, the therapist must be ready to explore the extent to which the child's work triggers or evokes their thoughts and feelings about their own childhood and parenting experiences. Supervision is critical in providing opportunities to understand the therapist's unexamined thoughts and feelings in treatment and reduce the likelihood of its interference with the treatment. For example, a therapist may become activated by a perceived lack of empathy in understanding some challenging behaviours in their child. The therapist's experience with the parent, coupled with the therapist's own childhood experiences, will shape the therapist's view of the parent and ability to work with the parent. Examining the therapist's experiences during supervision allows the therapist to clarify their own experience separately from their understanding of the parent.

Supervisors have the added responsibility of being aware of these potential dynamics between the therapist and the clients, recognising the therapist's vulnerability in sharing and discussing the emotions that are activated in work, and creating a safe space for the therapist to examine the potential impact of them on the therapeutic work. Ann Horne (see 'On finding a voice: thoughts on the role of supervisor', Chapter 1) supports the use of transference and countertransference in working with children but cautions that supervision should prioritise the therapist's need to find their voice over seeking a 'right way'.

Supervisors hold a tension between knowledge of technique and the importance of the therapeutic process. Several authors take up this issue (Martin Daltrop, Chapter 5; Evrinomy Avdi, Chapter 4; Iris Gibbs, Chapter 9). For Avdi, one must balance research rigour with finding one's research voice. In situations like those referenced by Daltrop and Janine Sternberg (Chapter 2), agency requirements and adherence to training shaped by a competency framework can conflict with a more process-oriented approach. Child therapists in service agencies are responsible for responding to urgent matters in the child's home or school.

Furthermore, therapists may feel pressured by parents, teachers and case management supervisors in the child's ecosystem to focus on measurable outcomes. Supervisors can bring their own experiences of being supervised or take an adaptive disposition towards the diverse work settings and cultures one may encounter. Ultimately, supervisors can be instrumental in helping therapists respond to the child's ecosystem while keeping the child's needs as a focus of the treatment.

While there are many more dimensions of the supervisory relationship to explore, one more, in particular, should be highlighted here. Supervisors must create environments where the supervisee is receptive to feedback about the therapeutic process. Supervisors can offer corrective instructions balanced by the possibility that the therapist may feel criticised. Ben Yeo emphasises the dichotomy in the supervisor's role between creating a space for reflection and that 'space' becoming anxiety-provoking for the supervisee ('Feel the force: the experience of a supervisee on the child and adolescent psychoanalytic psychotherapy training',

Chapter 3). Some therapeutic processes re-created in the session elude the therapist's awareness when working with children. Supervisors are best positioned to observe these unconscious processes by monitoring the therapist's reports of experiences in the session that are particularly challenging. Horne points out that 'doing' child psychotherapy is not a question of following rigid rules. As Anna Freud noted, it is simply the adaptation of psychoanalytic principles to work with children. The use of transference and countertransference, Horne finds to be central to this. For example, a therapist may share with the supervisor an experience of emotional response outside the therapist's usual demeanour or a particular counter-transference response to the child or parent that caught the therapist's attention and warrants further exploration. Working with children brings to the forefront the therapist's own childhood experiences. The therapist views the parent and child through the therapist's own experiences – conscious and unconscious. Supervision can provide a safe space for reflection and collaboration that helps the therapist consider the perspectives of the child, the parent and the therapist's thoughts and feelings in working with the child.

In closing, the book represents a diversity of thought, perspectives and settings encountered in supervisory relationships. An essential lens for the reader to adopt includes the child's ecosystem, the supervisor's multidimensional matrix and external and internal factors between the therapist and supervisor embodied in the supervisory relationship. Beyond all, I echo the sentiments of Ann Horne, who encourages us to support the therapist's self-discovery of their voice and therapeutic understanding.

Flight Path

She'll settle on your shoulder if you let her, be there
when you need her and sometimes when you don't, helping
you to listen and to think; a shape-shifter, you picture her
as bird – wise owl, incisive corvid, mischievous macaw.

As owl she's unruffled and reflective, clearsighted
even in the dark, sensing movements in the shadows,
alert to the smallest signs of change. *Pay attention,*
she urges, *attend to what attention brings.*

As corvid she's inquisitive, sharp billed, quick-witted,
cocks her head repeatedly, listens as you speak, tweaks
your ear occasionally to signal you to stop. *Be curious,*
she urges, *honest curiosity will bring your work to life.*

When she's macaw, she's loud and full of laughter, flying
off your shoulder to the floor to play; she enjoys herself,
unselfconscious with the toys. *Be playful,* she urges,
play's the way we know ourselves, the way we grow.

Take the time to truly wonder, they all chorus,
with the child and with yourself; practise patience,
learn how to sit and wait. Then they fly off to roost,
leave you wondering what will happen next.

And in those quiet, calm moments of your own,
you hear a different voice, at first uncertain,
but growing stronger like a song, and you know it
as your own voice, flying now and fully-fledged.

(Diana Cant)

Introduction

Deirdre Dowling and Julie Kitchener

Supervision is woven into the structures and processes of child and adolescent psychotherapy training and ongoing professional development. Within the National Health Service (NHS) and in private practice child psychotherapists' supervision skills are sought and much valued by colleagues from other disciplines, as well as in schools, fostering agencies and residential settings. Yet, while a plethora of books and papers on clinical supervision have appeared in the past two decades, these have been written by those working in related professions and in adult psychoanalysis, psychotherapy and counselling. Child psychotherapists have remained unusually silent, even though we are subject to the same ethical and professional demands and constraints. *Supervision in a Changing World: Reflections from Child Psychotherapy* sets out to redress the balance. It is the eighth in the Independent Psychoanalytic Approaches with Children and Adolescents series, and marks four decades since Anne Hurry and her colleagues established the Independent child and adolescent psychotherapy training at the British Association of Psychotherapists. Now the Independent Psychoanalytic Child and Adolescent Psychotherapy Association at the British Psychotherapy Foundation (IPCAPA at the bpf), the training has grown considerably and continues to produce graduates who are grounded in both classical and object relations approaches, and rooted in Independent thinking, theory and technique.

Supervision in a Changing World explores the ways in which a child psychotherapist's perspective can enliven and enrich the debate around the theory and practice of supervision, and how this, in turn, can help clinicians, patients and their families. Specifically, it asks what a child and adolescent psychotherapist can bring to our understanding of contemporary supervision and the supervisory relationship in the mental health, social work and childcare professions. With contributions from leading practitioners, some with experience spanning several decades, others more newly qualified, the book covers a range of issues that are key to child psychotherapy supervision. These include ethical considerations, the interplay between the supervisee and supervisor experience, the tensions and complexities of service supervision and of working with trauma, the role of process notes and report writing and of research supervision, supervising

DOI: 10.4324/9781003297604-1

work with children and adolescents with disabilities (and dealing with disabled networks), supervising colleagues in different settings and countries, group supervision and the training school perspective on supervision. Throughout, the contributors draw on their clinical and supervisory experience, describing their approach to the work and bringing their individual insights. Nonetheless, certain unifying themes emerge: how to provide a 'holding space' for the inevitable tensions and anxieties, supervision as a transitional experience and the importance of creativity and curiosity, enabling the supervisee to develop his/ her own 'voice', working with difference and recognising the impact of power relationships, as well as the implications of 'remote' supervision.

The book has been compiled at a time of significant global health and sociopolitical challenge, forcing organisations and individual practitioners to become increasingly innovative and adaptable, to re-evaluate previous conscious and unconscious assumptions around diversity and the dynamics of power that inform the delivery of training and professional practice. Supervision is at the heart of that challenge. We aim to show that, while not unique to the profession, the Independently minded child and adolescent psychotherapist's capacity to recognise the developmental as well as the disruptive potential of unconscious processes, to negotiate the tension between responsibility and creativity, between respect for expertise and the ability to question are qualities not only essential to therapeutic work with children but also to supervision in a changing world.

Behind this, of course, lies a broader question: what exactly does inform the child psychotherapist's thinking on supervision? Here, Deirdre Dowling and Julie Kitchener offer a brief overview of key thinkers who have influenced their approach to supervision and that of many contributors to this book.

Thinking and rethinking…

Deirdre Dowling

Thinking and rethinking, learning and relearning, is a continual process in the growth of a supervisor. It is hard to pinpoint the key influences out of many that have an impact on the changing psychoanalytic approaches, and sociopolitical developments. However, there are core ideas that have been crucial in shaping my thinking as a supervisor in the Independent tradition.

Michael Parsons writes:

> You cannot teach a child to grow up and you cannot teach someone to be a psychoanalyst: it is a question of helping them to become one.
>
> (Parsons 2014: 205)

I would agree, but providing a facilitating environment for this *becoming* to happen is crucial. Supervising new trainees reminds me of the agonising doubt I experienced when learning to offer therapy to very troubled children, who appear to respond so slowly to the therapeutic approach. Isca Salzberger-Wittenberg empha-sises the importance of containment to hold students though the pain of learn-ing anew:

> The task of the teacher may be thought of as resembling the parental function: that is to act as a temporary container for the excessive anxiety of his students at points of stress. It will mean he will experience in himself some of the mental pain connected with learning and set an example of maintaining curiosity in the face of chaos, love of truth in the face of the terror of the unknown and hope in the face of despair.
>
> (Wittenberg 1983: 60)

In his chapter in this book, Ben Yeo (Chapter 3) writes about his need for contain-ment when faced with this early self-doubt and then his growing confidence as he goes through the training and finds his own voice. Janine Sternberg (Chapter 2) describes the holding function of the Independent training she led, with its inter-connecting strands of teaching theory, supervision and developing practice skills. I recall from teaching at the Independent Psychoanalytic Child and Adolescent Psychotherapy Association (IPCAPA) training school, the warm encouraging atmosphere that is part of this rigorous training which helps the therapists begin to develop confidence in themselves.

One of the skills I have learnt as their intensive case supervisor is to respond sensitively to the changing needs of the developing child therapist trainees as they progress through the training. The necessary containment of trainees in the first two years moves to a more collaborative approach with the third- and fourth-year stu-dents, where ideas and techniques are explored together to shape our understanding of a child. The final-year students have to discover their own style and develop confidence in their own understanding in preparation for taking up their role in postgraduate work, whether in a clinic or private work.

As Bernard Barnett (2012) warns, there is always the danger of imposing too strict a framework, which creates a passive dependency in the student and a harsh superego. The trainee can lose his/her spontaneity and freedom of thought in the process, feeling inferior to the teachers. Similarly, Ann Horne ([2006]/2019b: 140) cites the dangers of us feeling inhibited by the Great Child Psychotherapist in the Sky, our fantasy that there is a right way to do things, or else we will be open to criticism by others.

This might be particularly true of trainees from a minority culture if they feel isolated in the trainee group and do not feel free to voice their own differing experi-ences of life and ways of thinking. Yet their contribution brings the multiple per-spectives vital to understanding our young patients.

Helping supervisees find their own technique and therapeutic understanding is a key aspect of the Independent approach, as Ann Horne explores in Chapter 1, 'On finding a voice: thoughts on the role of supervisor'. Following Winnicott, this necessitates providing *a facilitating environment*, adapted to the needs of the therapist, that will support the trainee in finding his/her authentic voice. This would need to take into account the therapist's earlier experience of working with children, the social and cultural context of the therapy, as well as the particular strengths and vulnerabilities of the practitioner.

It is interesting to consider how we can encourage open-minded and spontaneous thought in our role as supervisors, particularly when we are in an assessing teaching role. A child psychotherapist in training is having to learn a new structure and way of thinking. Trainees are aware that the supervisor has a central role in assessing their skills, which can inhibit an open dialogue, especially in the early years of learning.

There are a few writers that I have found particularly helpful as guides in this task of encouraging development. Early on, I read Patrick Casement's book *On Learning from the Patient* (1985) where he emphasised the importance of listening to the feedback he received from his patients in shaping the direction of their therapeutic work together. From their responses to his 'conversation' with them, he discovered what helped and what hindered their search for meaning and recovery in psychotherapy. This theme is taken up by Michael Parsons (2007) in 'Raiding the inarticulate', where he talks about the importance of therapists developing their own internal analytic setting to guide them in moments of uncertainty. He suggests that this will be informed by close listening to the patient, both to their verbal and nonverbal communication, and to their (the therapist's) own countertransference response to the patient. The supervisor's role here would be to offer the therapists the space for reflection where they can recognise that growing internal understanding of the therapeutic task.

Thomas Ogden reminds us that supervision, like therapy, is co-created:

Dreaming up the patient in the supervisory session represents … the combined effort of the analyst and supervisor to bring to life in the supervision what is true to the analyst's experience of what is occurring at a conscious, pre-conscious, and unconscious level in the analytic relationship.

(Ogden 2009: 34)

Usually, the therapist takes a difficulty or uncertainty about their treatment of the patient to supervision. Ogden suggests that when we can help the therapist recognise those underlying emotional feelings that inform the discussion about a patient, they can recognise what is obstructing their flow of thinking.

Monica Lanyado (2018: 89) focuses on the supervisor's role in noting signs of change in the therapist's work with traumatised children, and the importance of bringing this to the attention of the therapist. She observes that frequently there are significant moments in the relationship between therapist and child, 'moments of meeting' (Stern *et al.*1998) that emerge in therapeutic work with traumatised children, often after a period of despair. Lanyado suggests that this can indicate that there has been an emotional development in the child that may have been missed by the therapist immersed in the process. She points out that the experience of working with trauma can interfere with the therapist's thinking capacity. The supervisor who is an observer, outside the intensity of the therapeutic relationship, but in touch with the feelings brought to supervision, may be aware of these subtle changes presaging a development in the child before the therapist.

Taking a wider perspective, as a supervisor I have been strongly influenced by my family therapy colleagues and their systemic approach to understanding the dynamics of family life.

Psychotherapists in the Independent tradition have always stressed the importance of recognising the impact of the child's developmental history and the family context. Families from different cultural traditions have faced a diversity of experiences, and the impact of poverty, class and migration heightens the need for us to be open to exploring the particular meaning of the child's emotional difficulties to their parents, extended family or carers. As Pamela Bartram discusses in Chapter 8, the experience of raising a child with learning disability or autism will also have a significant impact on the experience of parenting and family life. A systemic approach to the family can offer us, as psychotherapists, a way to think about these dynamic differences when we offer support to parents whose child is in difficulties.

In his book *The Child, the Family and the Outside World* Winnicott ([1964]/ 2000) emphasised the importance of thinking about children within the network of their relationships. Often, little attention is given to the supervision of parent work, although supportive work with parents is a significant part of the qualified child psychotherapist's role, particularly as there are unlikely to be the resources to offer parents therapeutic work in their own right. It can be challenging for the therapist to keep in mind the perspective of both the child and the parent, particularly when the parents' views are at odds with the therapist's view of the child's needs. But integrating these two worlds and finding a balance between them will be crucial in ensuring that change is possible in both aspects of the child's world, the inner and the outside world. Supervision can provide a space for child therapists to reflect on their often conflicting counter-transference responses to the child and the parents, and to find a way to protect their therapeutic work with the child, while helping parents recognise their contribution and role in helping the child with their difficulties.

Similarly, at an organisational level, Isabel Menzies Lyth's work on social systems and their defences against anxiety (1960) has been crucial in shaping my ideas about the importance of the health of institutions to the wellbeing of their clients and the quality of therapeutic work that it is possible to do there. Working first as a social worker, and then in the Family Service at the Cassel Hospital, West London Mental Health Trust, I saw at first hand the interactive nature of the different systems at work in any organisation, and the importance of a reflective space for individuals and teams, at every level, to look at their role in the organisation. This helps to alleviate the damaging splits and tensions that can so easily happen when a team is in conflict, or an institution is under stress.

In my supervision of experienced psychotherapists who know the fundamentals of practice, I may spend as much time exploring the impact of institutional stresses on the therapist's capacity to think and contain the therapy as I will on the clinical material. This was particularly important during the pandemic, when the closure of clinics and schools and then their reopening in a fragmented state left the therapist struggling to find the containment needed to work effectively and to argue for what the individual child and family need. Maintaining a fine balance between focusing on the child's internal and external world, the therapist's emerging sense of direction and my own perspective as a supervisor is one of the interesting challenges of this role.

Framing and reframing

Julie Kitchener

In a playground at the top of the hill behind my house there is a notice that reads: 'Children must be supervised at all times.' At the bottom of the hill there is a second playground. Here the notice reads: 'Children must be supervised by a responsible adult.' I have no idea how many people read these signs. Certainly not the children who play there, though they will, inevitably, experience their effects, freighted as they are with contemporary anxiety about how we create 'safe spaces' for our children (and keep them out of mischief) while allowing them the freedom to explore and develop.

There is an obvious parallel here with the significance of the psychoanalytic frame. 'If we enter a theatre, a place of worship or a children's playground,' Michael Parsons suggests, 'we cross a boundary which tells us that the reality we are going to meet on the inside works differently from the reality outside' (Parsons 2007:1442).

However, the difference in the wording between the notice in the playground at the top of the hill and that at the bottom also encapsulates something of psychoanalysis's troubled relationship with supervision – the push and pull between anxious, autocratic surveillance and attentive, authoritative presence.

Michael Balint highlighted this tension more than 70 years ago. In his critique of psychoanalytic training and supervision, 'On the psycho-analytic training system', he challenged the prevalence of what he called 'unconscious and uncontrolled super-ego intropression', the result of an institutional approach that encouraged submissiveness to 'a strong paternal authority "to instruct and admonish"'. Instead, he argued, the aim of a psychoanalytic training should be 'building up a strong ego which shall be both critical and liberal at the same time' (Balint 1948: 167–171).

I came across this paper of Balint's in the early days of my training. Not, I should say, on a seminar reading list, but from a reference in a 2005 paper by Patrick Casement that was doing the rounds among trainees at the time, intriguingly entitled 'The Emperor's clothes: some serious problems in psychoanalytic training'. Casement, like Balint, addressed the flaws he saw in psychoanalytic training institutions. He decried the infantalisation of trainees ('candidates') through a dogmatic approach to supervision that dismantled trainees' thinking and stunted their emerging ways of working (Casement 2005: 1151), as well as what he called 'wild analysis in committee' – the tendency to evaluate (and pathologise) trainees' progress on the basis of their character rather than competence (1144). Casement's paper piqued the latent outrage of a new but mature trainee struggling with the transition from experienced professional to fledgling child and adolescent psychotherapist. Little had changed, it suggested, since Kernberg had been prompted to write his searing parody 'Thirty methods to destroy the creativity of psychoanalytic students'. Recommendation 27: 'refer ... back to the couch' (Kernberg 1996: 1038).

These criticisms were aimed at the adult institutions. However, child psychotherapy trainings, as we know from the Controversial Discussions in the 1940s through the 'controversial discussions without the discussion' (Horne [2006]/ 2019a: 14) of the late 1960s, are not immune to factionalism and polarising allegiances – the hallmarks, as Balint saw it, of 'super-ego intropression'. We no longer think in terms of 'control analysis', or debate whether a candidate's training analyst should double up as training case supervisor, and we would be shocked if, as happened to D W Winnicott, our supervisor (in his case, Melanie Klein) pressed to supervise our analysis of her son (he successfully resisted) (Phillips 1988: 47). Nonetheless, questions of power and accountability remain, especially in a training setting where supervisors' reports form part of the assessment process (see Deirdre Dowling above and Janine Sternberg, Chapter 2). Supervision, I learned from Balint, Kernberg and Casement, is a serious business. If I had been imagining a future supervisor self, I would have known exactly the supervisor I did *not* want to become.

Only, when it came to it, my own experience of training supervision turned out to be rather different – enjoyable, even. By which I mean, the training school's reputation for baking aside, each of my individual supervisors and clinical seminar leaders embodied their own supervisory interpretation of Charles Rycroft's description of the analytic setting:

> This setting is itself a communication to the patient, since its details are all signs that the analyst intends taking up a certain attitude towards the patient, that he intends to listen to him, to concern himself with him without requiring the patient to be concerned with him, and to protect the contact between them from external interruption or distraction.
>
> (Rycroft 1956: 470)

Rycroft offered what were then radical insights into contextual and affective communication; ideas that continue to inform my thinking, both in the room with a child and in supervision. The aim, Ann Horne suggests, is to 'present an environment that is not overwhelming in its possibilities but definitely offering a curious, engaged "other"' ([2006]/2019a: 20), a provision that includes the 'playful presence' of the supervisor (Lanyado 2018).

In Chapter 10, Coretta Ogbuagu contests a model of supervision in which knowledge is transmitted from one wise head to another that is less so. Implicit in this is the idea of 'deskilling' – that the trainee or therapist's prior experience

and knowledge are somehow irrelevant or need to be replaced. The group analyst Farhad Dalal considers such assumptions 'a form of colonization' (2021: 12).
In contrast, Thomas Ogden suggests, 'The supervisor is responsible for creating
a frame that ensures the supervisee's freedom to think and dream and be alive
to what is occurring both in the analytic process and in the supervisory process'
(2005: 1269). Ogden's co-creative process recognises the inevitable power differential between supervisor and supervisee, but relies on responsible, facilitating
authority, rather than omniscient authoritarianism. Arguably, this authority derives
from what Michael Parsons describes as 'the analyst's internal analytic setting'.
A secure internal frame, Parsons maintains, 'allows flexibility in the external setting' (2007: 1441). In supervision, this might mean responding to the difference
between the needs of a trainee and a qualified therapist, between clinical and
research supervision, individual or group, or indeed supervision. Evrinomy Avdi
notes this creative tension between internal security and external flexibility in her
chapter on the role of research supervisor (Chapter 4).

Viewed from a co-creative perspective, the question of what constitutes knowledge (and who 'owns' what knowledge) becomes more fluid. Freud, who had
little to say on the matter of supervision (Leader 2010: 229), did, however, make
the point that what goes on in an analysis can be known to others only through
'hearsay' (Freud [1915]/1916: 42). This reality alone undermines assumptions of
omniscience, even when parallel processing of transference and countertransference within the supervisory relationship forms part of the work. Knowledge,
Farhad Dalal argues, is an emergent property within well-functioning supervision;
'matters arising', he and his colleague call their peer supervisions (2021: 16). My
own understanding of psychotherapy supervision has evolved, and continues to
evolve, in much the same way: emerging from my experience as supervisor and as
supervisee. This is how I have come to know the value of Sándor Ferenczi's notion
of tact, Winnicott's sense of timing, Enid Balint's ability to wait (see Parsons' 2009
distillation of these Independent approaches, as well as Ann Horne's 'On finding a
voice', Chapter 1).

Learning from experience can take surprising turns. A particular revelation was
the Weaving Thoughts approach developed by Norman and Salomonsson (2005).
Weaving Thoughts draws heavily on Wilfred Bion's theory of groups and was
introduced in my final-year clinical seminars by a senior child analyst from the
Anna Freud Centre (Independent training at its pluralistic, nondoctrinal best). It
is an approach I continue to find helpful with groups. In Weaving Thoughts, the
facilitator offers nothing other than clear, simple guidelines for participation and
comment – no therapeutic advice, no interpretations of the session material – with
the effect that presenter and peers are protected from negative group dynamics, and
clinical understanding develops from shared free associative processes.

This is supervision informed by Winnicott's 'organized non-interference'
(1950: 250), or Horne's 'actively taking great care' ([2006]2019a: 19). Most
IPCAPA graduates are familiar with Juliet Hopkins' evocation of her supervision
with Winnicott, approaching him as an 'over-awed' trainee and discovering that,

far from dozing through their first meeting, as she had suspected, he had been listening intently.

> There was nothing doctrinal about his views. He never told me what to do or say. He listened with closed eyes and then shared his thoughts, letting me see how he played freely with alternative ideas and encouraging me to do the same.
>
> (Hopkins 1996a: 20–21)

An irresistibly humane and democratic model of supervision.

Such comforting aspirations carry their own risks, for both supervisor and supervisee. There is a fine line between emulation and idealisation, and those of us who think of ourselves as, say, Winnicottians, find we need to tread carefully. As Ann Horne cautions, idealisation 'tends all too speedily to be followed by institutionalisation' ([2006]/2019a:13). Independents, whatever their conscious intent, are as susceptible as anyone to transference and countertransference dynamics, to the 'related dangers of narcissism and idealisation' within the supervisory relationship (Lemma 2012: 456). Compounding these dynamics, perhaps more specifically for child psychotherapists, is the pull of maternal identifications. Despite object relations theory's fascination with mothering, little has been written about the issue of gender in supervision, as Ben Yeo notes in 'Feel the force', Chapter 3. Yet, in a field where most practitioners, and therefore supervisors, are women, the supervisor as good-enough mother is a seductive self-image.

'It seems,' wrote the late Mani Vastardis, one-time head of the British Association of Psychotherapists (BAP) child training and formidable clinical and service supervisor, 'that child psychotherapists fit very well – sometimes too well – the caring and mothering role unconsciously allocated to them … However, there is a danger lurking in this flattering assignment' (2009: 161). One aspect of this is the over-attunement that inhibits development and a healthy push to independence; the supervisory equivalent of 'the dangers and deprivations of too-good mothering' detailed by Juliet Hopkins in her startling reappraisal of her infant observation (1996b). This is a more subtle, yet equally stultifying, version of omniscient supervision: the hovering, helicopter parent, pre-emptively swooping in to scoop up and rescue. To paraphrase Winnicott, the therapist's creativity can be only too easily stolen by a supervisor who knows too much (1971: 67) – who can, for example, 'see' what the therapist is trying to achieve or what the patient is communicating, who 'foresees' possibilities and pitfalls in the therapeutic work. 'You have to risk playing some wrong notes', a piano teacher once told me, 'or the right notes just won't sound right.'

Paradoxically, Vastardis seems to be saying, child psychotherapists can become too focused on an ideal of environmental provision, too primarily preoccupied with the therapeutic dyad. As result, she warns, 'We could risk seeing ourselves – and more importantly and dangerously, in these difficult times, risk being seen by others – as standing above the fray.' How much more difficult the times have become since Vastardis wrote those words. Martin Daltrop in this book (Chapter 5), addresses the real-world challenges faced by the CAMHS supervisor, positioned, as Vastardis puts it, 'at the interface between an external, political world and an internal psychological and emotional one' (2009: 161).

Recent events have forced the child psychotherapy profession, along with our adult analytic colleagues, to re-evaluate and reframe our position at this interface, as Teresa Bailey takes up in Chapter 7. It is odd that it has taken the Covid crisis, the Black Lives Matter movement and the campaigns around sexuality and gender to remind us of questions of identity, power and exclusion, given that psychoanalytic theory holds potential insights into the unconscious forces at play in these issues. Feminists claimed the personal as political half a century ago, with writers such as Jacqueline Rose, Dorothy Dinnerstein, Nancy Chodorow, Hélène Cixous interrogating as well as contributing to psychoanalytic thought. And before them, Frantz Fanon identified the effects of colonialism on racial consciousness, his now classic texts, *Black Skin, White Masks* ([1952]1967) and *The Wretched of the Earth* ([1961]1963), anticipating contemporary critiques of the political and psychic workings of racism.

This apparent neglect of 'the outside inside', the fact that some people, as Christopher Bollas puts it, suffer 'overdetermination from the outside' (2018: 36) is particularly shocking given the communities we serve (see, for example, Pamela Bartram, Chapter 8, and Iris Gibbs, Chapter 9), as well as the diversity of most multidisciplinary teams in CAMH and social care services. Psychoanalytic Super Vision, it seems, has been doggedly unseeing, whether this be through rigid institutional insistence on psychoanalytic 'truths', or what the Jungian analyst Helen Morgan calls 'a cheerful self-imposed blindness' (2008: 38). Morgan and Dalal are among a growing number of adult analysts contributing to the previously neglected discussion about the role of supervision in tackling issues of diversity and exclusion. As Morgan points out (2008: 39–40), these are not easy matters to play with – as therapists or supervisors: a significant challenge for anyone schooled in a tradition that sets so much store by playing – particularly those of us working with children.

Which brings us back to the playground ... Could there be a clue here about child psychotherapists' apparent reticence in writing about supervision? We aim to get alongside the children we work with, to see the world from their point of view. Prone as we may be to maternal identifications, the identification with the child can be stronger: supervision, like parent work, is for the grown-ups. This book, we hope, proves otherwise; more, that Independent psychoanalytic child psychotherapy has a unique contribution to make in the field of supervision. Child psychotherapists are not children, but they do spend a lot of time with them. It was, after all, a child who saw through the Emperor's new clothes.

References

Balint, M (1948) On the psycho-analytic training system. *The International Journal of Psychoanalysis 29*: 163–173.

Barnett, B (2012) Psychoanalytic learning, training, teaching and supervision. In P Williams, J Keene and S Dermen (eds.) *Independent Psychoanalysis Today* London: Karnac.

Bollas, C (2018) *Meaning and Melancholia: Life in the Age of Bewilderment* Abingdon: Routledge.

Casement, P (1985) *On Learning from the Patient* London: Tavistock Publications.

Casement, P (2005) The Emperor's clothes: some serious problems in psychoanalytic training. *The International Journal of Psychoanalysis 86*: 1143–1160.

Dalal, F (2021) The ethics of supervision: reciprocity, emergence and prefiguration. *Group Analysis* Sage Journals https://doi.org/10.1177/05333164211050756.

Fanon, F ([1952]1967) *Black Skin, White Masks* (*Peau Noire, Masques Blancs*) London: Penguin Classics.

Fanon, F ([1961]1963) *The Wretched of the Earth* (*Les Damnés de la Terre*) Harmondsworth: Penguin Books.

Freud, S ([1915]/1916) *Lecture One. Introductory Lectures in Psychoanalysis*, Volume *1* Harmondsworth: Pelican Freud Library.

Hopkins, J (1996a) From baby games to let's pretend: the achievement of playing. *Journal of the British Association of Psychotherapists 31*: 20–27.

Hopkins, J (1996b) The dangers and deprivations of too-good mothering. *Journal of Child Psychotherapy 22* (*3*): 407–422.

Horne, A ([2006]/2019a) The Independent position in psychoanalytic psychotherapy with children and adolescents: roots and implications. In A Horne *On Children Who Privilege the Body: Reflections of an Independent Psychotherapist* London: Routledge.

Horne, A ([2006]/2019b) Interesting things to say to children – and why. In A Horne *On Children Who Privilege the Body: Reflections of an Independent Psychotherapist* London: Routledge.

Kernberg, F (1996) Thirty methods to destroy the creativity of psychoanalytic candidates. *The International Journal of Psychoanalysis 77*: 1031–1040.

Lanyado, M (2018) The playful presence of the therapist: 'antidoting' defences in the therapy of a late-adopted adolescent boy. In M Lanyado *Transforming Despair to Hope: Reflections on the Psychotherapeutic Process with Severely Neglected and Traumatised Children* Abingdon: Routledge.

Leader, D (2010) Some thoughts on supervision. *British Journal of Psychotherapy 26* (*2*): 228–241.

Lemma, A (2012) Some reflections on the 'teaching attitude' and its application to teaching about the use of the transference: a British view. *British Journal of Psychotherapy 28* (*4*): 454–473.

Menzies Lyth, I (1960) The functioning of social systems as a defence against anxiety: a report on a study of the nursing service of the general hospital. In I Menzies Lyth *Containing Anxiety in Institutions: Selected Essays* Volume *1* London: Free Association Books.

Morgan, H (2008) Issues of 'race' in psychoanalytic psychotherapy: whose problem is it anyway? *British Journal of Psychotherapy 24* (*1*): 34–49.

Norman, J and Salomonsson B (2005) 'Weaving thoughts': a method for presenting and commenting psychoanalytic case material in a peer group. *The International Journal of Psychoanalysis 86*: 1281–1298.

Ogden, T (2005) On psychoanalytic supervision. *The International Journal of Psychoanalysis 86* (*5*): 1265–1280.

Ogden, T (2009) *Rediscovering Psychoanalysis: Thinking and Dreaming, Learning and Forgetting* The New Library of Psychoanalysis. London and New York: Routledge.

Parsons, M (2007) Raiding the inarticulate: the internal analytic setting and listening beyond countertransference. *The International Journal of Psychoanalysis 88* (6): 1441–1456.

Parsons, M (2009) An Independent theory of clinical technique. *Psychoanalytic Dialogues 19* (3): 221–236.

Parsons, M (2014) Forming an identity, reflections on psychoanalytic training. In *Living Psychoanalysis: From Theory to Experience* The New Library of Psychoanalysis. Hove: Routledge.

Phillips, A (1988) *Winnicott* Cambridge, MA: Harvard University Press.

Rycroft, C (1956) The nature and function of the analyst's communication to the patient. *The International Journal of Psychoanalysis 37*: 469–472.

Stern, D N, Sander, L W, Nahum, J P, Harrison, A M, Lyons-Ruth, K, Morgan, A C, Bruschweiler-Stern, N and Tronick, E Z (1998) Non-interpretive mechanisms in psychoanalytic therapy. The 'something more' than interpretation. *The International Journal of Psychoanalysis 79*: 903–921.

Vastardis, G (2009) 'You are paid to be a nuisance': tensions in the role of a clinician-manager. In A Horne and M Lanyado (eds.) *Through Assessment to Consultation* Hove: Routledge.

Winnicott, D W (1950) The meaning of the word democracy. In *Home is Where We Start From* London: Penguin.

Winnicott, D W ([1964/2000]) *The Child, the Family and the Outside World* London: Penguin.

Winnicott, D W (1971) Playing: the search for the self. In *Playing and Reality* London: Penguin.

Wittenberg, I S (1983) The emotional aspects of learning. In I S Wittenberg, G Henry and E Osborne (eds.) *The Emotional Experience of Learning and Teaching* London: Karnac.

Part 1

The supervisor's task

Chapter 1

On finding a voice

Thoughts on the role of supervisor

Ann Horne

Amongst the many by-products of the experience of working and supervising during the Covid-19 pandemic of 2020–2022 has been a heightened recognition of the vital importance of supervision, of its essential place in our practice. When the Association of Child Psychotherapists (ACP) in the latter part of 2020 piloted a series of online reflective groups for supervisors, it did so appreciating that the holding and containment these would offer could be replicated and made available to even more supervisees. It was a timely and valued initiative. Psychoanalytic trickle-down proved to be genuine, not the myth of economic theory, and participation in ACP-organised supervision groups was then offered to the entire membership. The chance to share fear and anxiety, creativity and curiosity and the seeming enactment of internal terrors in the real environment was grasped with relief and demand grew for further opportunities.

That this took place in groups was also important – it did not breach established individual supervisor-supervisee dyads or peer group supervisions but added a further dimension of listening, sharing, encountering a wider thinking world of colleagues, when many were isolating and isolated away from contact. We met colleagues whom we had never met before, certainly never entered into discussion with, and found we were thinking and engaging across boundaries of geography, training schools and theoretical perspectives with, frequently, relieved recognition and insight. Contact with others as they engaged with new demands, and contact with other ways of thinking and perceiving, both came high on the list of what was most appreciated. This reaffirmation of supervision and the sense of agency and creativity it can bring mattered.

Starting out ...

I find offering supervision to colleagues slightly embarrassing: I prefer to call it consultation as we are equals and I can feel my ears turn pink when asked. Our meetings become, then, more times of free associations to the material and the history, and times for joint reflection.

With trainees, on the other hand, there are certain approaches that I find helpful and some issues which should be addressed to help their future therapist-selves grow. Most of this chapter focuses on these.

DOI: 10.4324/9781003297604-3

We *can* see this supervisory process as hierarchical, one's years of knowledge and experience often denoting whether one is ready to supervise or not and whether that is supervision of colleagues, trainees or other professions. This is how it was when I trained: certainly, experience and further training were essential before one was invited to be a supervisor of trainee child psychotherapists. It required three years of work post-qualification, writing up a further supervised intensive case and providing notes on every case one had ever worked with at any frequency (80+ children and families), plus attending workshops on supervision, before applying to the British Association of Psychotherapists (BAP) to be admitted as a Senior Member. This was to grow into what became a very healthy annual course on supervision and we have Rosalie Joffe to thank for developing it.

But supervision that offers psychoanalytic understanding was and is made available to those who work with children in many settings. I recall being invited to meet fortnightly with the teaching group of a small school for children with emotional and behavioural difficulties, running a reflective group, in my first full child psychotherapy post, in return for being allowed to park in their playground when I went to work in the nearby hospital out-patient child psychiatry department (I viewed this as a very fulsome repayment) – such experiences of consultation are now expected to be gained by trainees during training.

Yet prior to entering training, providing consultation and supervision may well have been part of the work of many candidates. When applicants become trainees, we must not diminish the experience they bring, claiming that they are now expected to learn to offer something 'better' or 'deeper' (hierarchical again). The psychologist who brings cognitive understanding or the social worker who is at ease with systemic thinking have a breadth to offer that can only add to our own psychoanalytic perspective. And both may well have spent years teaching and supervising within their original professions. To become, then, the least experienced junior can be infantilising. It is one of the tasks of supervisors to see the wholeness of the person they are working with, what strengths and experience they bring as well as what development they need to make. It has not always been so: we have not always managed this well.

What might be some of the overarching aims of supervision?

Briefly described, the aim of therapy is to engage with the child or young person in exploring anxieties and defences that inhibit normal psychological development and functioning, and to work jointly towards the development of age-appropriate functioning and defences. In supervision, we hope to support the supervisee in gaining a fuller understanding of the patient and in developing /strengthening techniques that allow attunement to the patient, assist the application of psychoanalytic understanding to work with the patient and promote resilience and reflection in the therapist. For the supervisor of child work, the recognition that development is back on course as much as it can be is an important indicator to teach the trainee.

This list is neither universal nor exclusive…

Right?

I do not hold an institutionalised view of what is 'correct' or 'right' practice that I feel must then be passed on to trainees and supervisees. It seems to me that this would necessitate passing on the burden of an impossible superego. The need to get things 'right' (indeed the belief that such a possibility exists) contradicts the essential Independent view that analysis and supervision entail a *process between* two people (not something that is *done* by one to another as a doctor might lance a boil) – and one that is unique to each working dyad and essentially co-created. The supervisor is in a good position to contest the sense of a right way, that one way which must be replicated; rather we seek to foster in the supervisee a sense of curiosity as to how and why things happen in these spaces between therapist and patient. Supervision is (as Michael Parsons has said about becoming a psychoanalyst) a process that is developmental rather than didactic (Parsons 2014). Supervising my adolescent intensive training case, Anne Hurry[1] used to say to me: 'Now that was interesting! Why did you say/do that?' and I felt really invited to be curious about what was going on and to think it through with her. There was not a right way that I had got wrong; there was an interaction between the child and me that should be explored.

Anna Freud puts it well when she comments that child psychoanalysis is simply the adaptation of psychoanalytic principles to work with children: "There is no absolute psychoanalytic technique for use with children, but rather a set of analytic principles which have to be adapted to specific cases" (Sandler, Kennedy and Tyson 1980: 199).

I *do* have fairly firm ideas on what is *appropriate* – and you may well think I am a trifle pedantic in this. When I was a student, training to become a child and adolescent psychotherapist while latterly managing a multi-professional team in a Child Guidance Unit, many aspects of training were still quite formal. Indeed, some could be viewed as rigid. I recall one of my tutors describing, in her own training in another school, seeing children up to five times weekly dressed in the same clothes each time, and my wondering whether this really had more to do with dogma than anything else. Equally, trainee psychotherapists often stood like statues in waiting rooms, neither speaking nor nodding to their small patients and carers, waiting to be seen and followed to therapy rooms, afraid that a transference might be damaged were they to be found to be in any way proactive or individualistic. This always seemed a perversion of reality, an attempt to be a blank screen that is quite destined to fail. For some children, it is essential that we arrive in the waiting room as live objects whose bearing indicates that being alive and present and wishing to engage with them matters, children perhaps who cannot hold in mind an object who might be constant, or who need to be claimed again at each encounter; for others, we must observe whether we are allowed to be alive. Supervisees thus have to be helped to use their feelings, learn about the counter-transference, pause and consult it, from the moment of engaging with their child patients, and to take a moment to reflect on what this shows them. Equally, it can make all the difference to some children and parents/carers to give a nod of acknowledgement or word of greeting to the latter before going off with the child. One approach does not fit all – but we need to know how our flexibility might be construed and why. How we dress, how we create and inhabit space, is open to consideration in the light of the uniqueness of the relationship between *this* therapist and *this* child – what is appropriate with one child will not be with another, and supervisees will value being able to think this through; but there is no one way to be. When I worked in Southwark and Greenwich, I would dress fairly smartly in jackets and skirts – as I always had in every job in the past. When I moved to the Portman Clinic, I found myself beginning to wear trousers, aware of the multiply abused young people I saw who struggled with what might be felt to be seductive, and which might distract them into the need to defend against it. It varies with the patient and our understanding of that child and his/her history.

Perhaps Winnicott's comment that 'I aim at being myself and behaving myself' in his paper 'The aims of psychoanalytical treatment' (Winnicott 1962: 166) points to the possibility of finding an ego-syntonic way of being that does not impose on the patient.

Finding a voice

This seemingly light remark about 'being myself' resonates with the issue of finding one's own voice. Working within the framework of a moral and ethically humane stance aiming to make unconscious processes conscious and defences more tolerable and appropriate, we hope to help the supervisee find and develop his/her own style, learning to be adaptive to the rhythm of the patient. This is particularly important when we supervise for several training schools: if we see the supervisory process as drawing out a 'therapist true self', we must take care not to impose only our own selves.

The process of therapy, in Winnicott's experience, is akin to that of good-enough mother and growing infant, providing attunement, holding, resilience and creating space for development. It is, then, not too great a step to view the process of supervision in similar terms: that the supervisee comes to a relationship where the supervisor provides a space for thought, development and reflection. We aim therefore to be good enough. There is one particularly important aspect of this. Consider Freud's concept of the ego ideal – the growing sense in the toddler of who he would like to be and, more vitally, how he would like the world to view him. It is a developmental achievement after the narcissistic, more brittle stage of the ideal ego, rigid and vulnerable, founded in fantasy and not reality, itself a bridge between the loss of narcissism and the arrival of reality. When we fall short of our ego ideal, we feel shame. I have never found humiliation – which seeks to cause shame – to be helpful, not in teaching nor in therapy nor in child development. If we teach with a style that can undermine and humiliate, we will never help to structure the growing professional ego, nor support a psychotherapist-ego-ideal into maturity; rather, we may encourage defences against shame in our supervisees. I do feel strongly about this, having encountered colleagues in the wider profession who clearly had such experiences in their trainings. Again, it assumes that we can fall short of a 'right' way and fail. In a sense, if we do not attend to the 'ego ideal' of the supervisee, we may be promulgating an approach that insists on the person supervised having to approximate to a 'mini-me', become a clone of a kind and so a false self.

It may sound simplistic but it *is* important to value the 'other' and difference. Often, we supervise colleagues from other disciplines who have no desire to become child psychotherapists but who do wish to reflect on their work with children and add further psychoanalytic understanding and approaches to their own repertoire. I have learned a great deal in discussions with Art Psychotherapists in supervision with me where the triangulation of patient/therapist/image offers yet another route to thought, and I have warm memories of one such therapist working exceptionally creatively with violent young men in a South London regional resource centre. Psychoanalytic thinking is *not* our personal game park – *qua* Strachey (1940) and the Freud family.

Just as there is no *right* way of being a therapist, so there is no right way of supervising and offering consultation. We all have, in our minds, the voices of those who supervised us, of those who analysed us, and are aware that we are still in relationships with them. Many remain creatively in our work; some less so. I remember listening to Joe Sandler speaking at the Anna Freud Centre (AFC) in Maresfield Gardens when I was a relatively young supervisor of trainees on the AFC training, and feeling startled and delighted when he stated that he still had conversations with both his analysts inside his head and – after a pause – 'I tell the first one off!' The same is true of supervisors …

This might indicate that in thinking about supervision we ought to include the concept of a good fit – in this, it is parallel to analysis. When I reflect on supervisions that I have sought post-qualification, I realise that I chose people who would enrich my technique, whom I knew I wanted to learn from. I think this is true of most of us as we age in the profession.

Containment without omnipotence

There seems to be a theme in the literature on supervision that comes under the heading of 'self-disclosure'. It concerns using one's counter-transference to the supervisee and articulating these feelings, particularly where projections from the patient whose treatment is being discussed are involved and influence the supervisor-trainee connection. Being able to reflect on this together is important, examining just what has got into our joint relationship from the combination of process and the material being presented.

But there is also a far simpler form of disclosure that can be very enabling, that involves what and how one learned oneself. We can so easily appear omniscient and omnipotent. The most useful example I have found to give trainees struggling with the drive to interpret is my own experience with my first training case, just over three years old, whose response to my continuing interpretations was a firm 'Shut up!' I remember taking the session to Rose Edgcumbe who quietly said, 'Listen to him!' I needed to hear that. It is important for supervisees to know that we *do* know how it feels – indeed, we still remember it 40 years later ... Anna Freud gives a lovely example:

> Long ago I reported the case of a little boy with severe anxiety symptoms. I had scarcely analysed the anxiety in one form when it appeared in another. Finally he said, "Do you think it is really sensible that you chase it around like that?"
>
> (Sandler, Kennedy and Tyson 1980: 183–184)

Her work is full of instances from her practice. These demystify, de-idealise and elucidate in the most helpful way. Indeed, those supervisors who stay in my own mind when I work – part of my internal repertoire –are those for whom being ideal-ised (hence institutionalised, I think) is utterly foreign: Anne Hurry, Adam Phillips and Anne Alvarez come first to mind.

Supervision of work with traumatised and especially sexually abused children necessitates a particular kind of containment for the trainee – not simply man-aging and understanding powerful counter-transference feelings (tough as this is) but also constantly helping supervisees keep developmental insult in mind while they contend with a range of primitive defence mechanisms and manoeu-vres (shouting, breaking boundaries by running around the clinic, re-enactment, singing at the top of the voice, kicking, spitting [that's the pits for me] and so on – although one might be driven to comment that such defences cannot really be lost to mind ...). For the child who has been treated as a part object, unseen by anyone with a protective eye, making distress public is one way of projecting shameful memory onto the therapist and of trying to engage an unseeing world. The experience can feel very threatening to any therapist, especially as it inev-itably contains a strong possibility of public exposure and humiliation. It really matters in such cases to be able to trust the detail of process records and to help supervisees learn that there is meaning in the activity, often meaning that can be elicited and elaborated with hindsight from the notes as well as understood from the process in (or out of) the therapy room. It helps them *anticipate* unbearable terror in their small patients. It also matters that they know that such cases chal-lenge us all; that attacks on thought and competence are part of necessary and desperate communication.

Here I think we can sometimes find differences in approach amongst the dif-ferent theoretical traditions and it is an area of supervising where I do always rec-ommend reading – especially on aggression and violence, where I like trainees to master Glasser, Winnicott and Anna Freud. It is imperative that they come to recog-nise when aggression is an expression of agency, perhaps never exercised before, a developmental achievement, or a defence against feared attack or humiliation. Developing the supervisee's capacity to respond creatively to defences is a central part of our role. That a child is terrified and so attacks a therapist (i.e. the attack is perceived as the defence that it is) allows a different perspective and response than thinking that the child is aggressive – innately so – and even psychopathic, a word that really should never be used of a child. This is such an important piece of learning and the support of supervisor – and theory – is essential.

Other areas I tend to emphasise

Privileging the counter-transference

I find the counter-transference is often the focus of my supervision and I find it to be the arena in which trainees mature into therapists as they grasp its full potency. It is also a main aspect of supervising – using one's counter-transference to the material, the child and the supervisee as one reflects on the supervision session. Theorists like Parsons (2014), Casement (1985) and Carpy (1989) are essential allies for those seeking to hone its use.

In this, we must *also* help our trainees learn to make use of their bodily counter-transference, of how the child makes us feel and our physical responses. Recognising these as relevant and being encouraged to bring them to supervision is helpful. Today we are much more open to learning from this; it is especially necessary when we are working with children whose insult is preverbal, who have recourse to body-based defences which can be enactments of early, unnamed, unprocessed feelings.

All psychotherapists may fear *they* may act (rather than reflect) when in the presence of a particular child and the defences and material that the child brings – and we may, in our counter-transference be alerted to this in the trainee. This can be true especially when we feel the force of the counter-transference, when our own feelings become hard to manage – feeling overwhelmed, paralysed or filled with rage and an internal urge to retaliate sadistically. The crushing nature of the life experiences of many children can also give rise to a defensive sentimentality in the therapist. It is important as supervisor to help the supervisee find that narrow perch where one feels and recognises the emotional impact on the child but does not tip into sentimentality. The former allows us to be open to the full force in the transference – and to make use of our counter-transference feelings; the latter excludes these and, as Winnicott states, 'is useless … as it contains a denial of hate' (Winnicott 1947: 202). It also denies the negative transference and the therapist who continues to rely on sentiment is no use as a clinician.

Creating space for thinking is vital and helping supervisees find that little island in the mind described by Casement (1985) as well as that space in the room really matters in supervision. Trainees may well need permission to say to a child, 'Look, I'm not sure what's happening here, so I'll just take a wee minute to have a think about it.' The intensity for the child of having an experience of being thought about is mirrored in the trainee when he/she can find that space and recognise its forcefulness and surprising impact – again, it is a process *between* the two.

Pace, timing, intimacy

Juliet Hopkins (1996) has written of Winnicott's supervision of her three-year-old training patient. I recommend this to all trainees as it emphasises not-doing, an important activity that should be compulsory to rehearse (remember my training patient and Rose Edgcumbe ...), or at least not doing what Juliet had been taught was psychoanalytic. The early work of the therapy involved naming affects, giving a child who had no words, but who acted and moved mightily, /her words to make sense of his feelings and reflecting back these and his/her actions. (Miss Freud would have recognised the appropriateness of this developmental psychoanalysis.) The pace of the work and the timing of when interpretation might be offered was the key, the therapist creating space where being known and so beginning to know oneself emotionally can be countenanced. When we are able as supervisors to create ourselves that space for reflection, a different place that exists in its own time with its own rhythm and pace, we let our trainees feel in turn what it is like to provide this for the child. It is a space, for the moment, out of time. Each patient-therapist duo has to find its own tempo, the therapist has to learn to recognise and be in tune with the rhythm of the patient. Equally each supervisor and trainee dyad finds its own cadence which the trainee can then draw on.

Intimacy is also an issue to explore with trainees, beginning with where does the child choose to sit or play. We tend to have analysts who sit in the same chair while we lie on the same couch: our models here may not be helpful ... (I realised that my analyst had a sense of humour when, at our initial meeting, I hesitated in the doorway and she said, 'Well, I usually sit here ...') When meeting a new child, I linger in the doorway and invite the child to sit where he/she would feel comfortable. This allows a big choice of space and distance and lets me sense what degree of closeness, intimacy or distance that child might manage. I then say, 'I think I'll sit here ...' and move to where *feels* best. I do encourage trainees to think about closeness and distance from their first encounters, then think through why their counter-transference feelings are telling them that and later to use this as one yardstick of a child's increasing security and development as the therapy continues. With so many abused and neglected patients today, the meaning of intimacy to any child matters greatly and it is a theme we must keep in mind and teach.

Gaze

During the recent pandemic, it was perhaps the frame of analysis that came to be tested initially – time, day and participants possibly remained the same but venue, journey, arrival and departure became very different. Those who carry out online or telephone therapies found themselves inundated with queries about best practice from colleagues inexperienced in these.

Early in the pandemic, Adam Gopnik interviewed analysts and therapists about their experiences of 'remote therapy' (Gopnik 2020). Most respondents expressed disquiet that so many people – especially in essential public services – were 'deferring trauma until it becomes impossible to repress', but following that major issue, their concerns centred in the main on gaze – on seeing and being seen. There are the glimpses of other lives lived more visibly; there is the close intensity of faces on a screen – 'I can see the tears, I can hear the cracks'; and there is one's own face and home background, shockingly distracting when first encountered, like a disturbing mirror. For me, it was the shock of seeing a bouncy terrier self, eager to contribute, swaying into and away from the screen in a (hopefully) exaggerated version of myself.

I was reminded of the need to consider how one is seen; but I was also reminded of the importance of gaze and of its being part of what we draw attention to in supervision. Gaze can attack, penetrate and shame; and it can contain, hold, and give assurance. We need to help our trainees learn the subtlety of this.

Taking a history

One final point: as Winnicott wrote, 'The essential thing is I do base my work on diagnosis' (Winnicott 1962: 169). I find it imperative to have a good history and I encourage supervisees to gather what information lies in their agencies about the child patient and his family. If there is sparse detail, this matters and may be a strong indication that the child has never been enabled to develop a sense of 'going on being', of developmental attainment, but may well simply survive by living in the moment. It is astonishing how often good information – especially the thoughts of foster carers – is available but has not been collated. It is important as so many of the children we now work with have been traumatised at early stages of develop-ment. This is not to decry the place of the 'state of mind assessment' when a one-off meeting with a child is used to gain insight into his/her functioning and expecta-tions of his/her objects. However, where what children *do* is what has brought them to the service, one needs to find the events and internalisations from the past that have formed the defences and created the triggers for their behaviours – and this is our main patient group today. Supervisor and trainee need to go over the contents of the assessment and history from time to time and will rediscover seemingly unknown – lost – information that, at later stages, helps make sense of the positions the child feels compelled to adopt.

Conclusion

Once we have settled into our role as supervisors, we find a freedom in engaging with another adult, creating a transitional space for thinking about a child. It's like being an auntie, not a parent – the responsibilities are different and opportunities exist for diverse discourses and ways of reflecting. It must be in the forefront of our minds that we are engaged in that 'developmental not didactic' process (Parsons 2014) – our trainees are growing into the kind of therapists they would wish to be, and their experience of us affects that and the kind of supervisors they will, in turn, become. And as with analysis there is no completed analysis, only an internalised process that the patient will draw on over the years, so we retain, internally, good supervisors to question and inform us as we continue to develop.

I leave the last words to Mani Vastardis, writing with Gail Phillips about their supervisory relationship:

> What seems to be important is for the supervisor, through her tact and empathy, to provide an environment in which play and 'dreaming up' (Ogden 2005) of the patient in the overlap between the therapeutic and the supervisory relationship becomes possible. This environment will hopefully maintain a feeling of space for unhurried thinking, for '*guided dreaming*', for occasionally 'having time to waste' ..., something which the supervisee will be seeking to safeguard in his own practice following qualification for the benefit of the therapeutic dyad.
>
> (Vastardis and Phillips 2012: 120, emphasis in original)

Note

1 Anne [Annie] Hurry established the then-BAP (now IPCAPA) child and adolescent psychotherapy training. A staff member of the Anna Freud Centre in Hampstead, she had additionally trained as an adult psychotherapist at the British Association of Psychotherapists and was a staff member at Brent Adolescent Centre.

References

Carpy, D V (1989) Tolerating the counter-transference: a mutative process. *International Journal of Psychoanalysis 70 (1)*: 287–294.

Casement, P (1985) *On Learning from the Patient* London and New York: Tavistock Publications.

Gopnik, A (2020) The new theatrics of remote therapy: how does treatment change when your patients are on a screen? *The New Yorker* 1 June.

Hopkins, J (1996) From baby games to let's pretend: the achievement of playing. *Journal of the British Association of Psychotherapists 31*: 20–28.

Ogden, T (2005) On psychoanalytic supervision. *International Journal of Psychoanalysis 86*: 1265–1280.

Parsons, M (2014) An Independent theory of clinical technique. *Psychoanalytic Dialogues 19*: 221–236.

Sandler, J, Kennedy, H and Tyson, R (1980) *The Technique of Child Psychoanalysis: Discussions with Anna Freud* London: The Hogarth Press and The Institute of Psychoanalysis.

Strachey, J (1940) Letter to Glover 23rd April. Quoted in E Rayner *The Independent Mind in British Psychoanalysis* London: Free Association Books 1991.

Vastardis, M and Phillips, G (2012) On psychoanalytic supervision: avoiding omniscience, encouraging play. In A Horne and M Lanyado (eds.) *Winnicott's Children* Hove and New York: Routledge.

Winnicott, D W (1947) Hate in the counter-transference. In *Collected Papers: Through Paediatrics to Psychoanalysis* London: Hogarth Press 1975.

Winnicott, D W (1962) The aims of psychoanalytical treatment. In *The Maturational Processes and the Facilitating Environment* London: The Hogarth Press 1965.

Chapter 2

What aids learning?

Thinking about supervision and
teaching from a training school's
perspective

Janine Sternberg

I am writing this chapter from the perspective of having been the Clinical Course
Director, usually known as Head of Training (HoT), of the Independent training
for child psychotherapists for the last eight years, and heavily involved in thinking
about and delivering the training for at least ten years before that.

There is so much to think about when considering teaching in general, and psychoanalytic education in particular. Kernberg's famous 1986 paper describes how
education within psychoanalytic institutions could be seen as profoundly unhelpful
and counterproductive. His describing psychoanalytic training as an 'educational
enterprise' (Kernberg 2018) was even thought of as strange when he first raised it.
He gathers much of his thinking in a 2021 paper in which he also makes a plea for
the psychoanalytic community to take a greater interest in neurobiology and other
ways of understanding both the mind and the body that have emerged in more
recent years. Slavin also points out that psychoanalytic and psychotherapy trainings have been traditionally 'insulated from the traditions of the academy' (Slavin
1997: 808): institutions have been private, self-regulating and not much given to
questioning.

Of course, I have been concerned with the learning journeys of child psychotherapy trainees in the UK in the first 20 years of the twenty-first century, and think
that the context is different from the one in which Kernberg was writing. When
looking back on his paper in 2018 he stated:

> So from this viewpoint, psychoanalysis – this treatment is a scientific procedure
> that can be learned and acquired ... the nature of the learning experience should
> be that of learning scientific skill. And implies therefore learning a technique,
> it's a highly specialized technical university setting. Plus, the stimulation of
> individual creativity, that has something to do with teaching of the arts. One can
> be inspired by one's teachers, which has to develop one's own style. So ideally,
> the education should have aspects of a university college, and an art school.
>
> (Kernberg 2018: page 2 of transcribed interview)

The 'university' model he propounds is indeed the wider context within which
we are operating, and qualification courses have become doctoral programmes,

DOI: 10.4324/9781003297604-4

acknowledging the depth and breadth of knowledge that qualified child psycho-therapists have. How have they attained this knowledge? In many different ways of course – through actively doing the work under supervision, through receiving academic teaching related to both theory relevant to the work and research activity and through completing academic assignments, which include taking exams and writing clinical papers. They also attain this knowledge through independent research, data gathering and using validated methodologies to analyse the data and shaping their findings into a coherent narrative. This all takes place over a four-year full-time programme that aims to produce thoughtful and skilled clinician-researchers.

Much child psychotherapy teaching is done in a non-didactic way, influenced by ideas such as Bion's (1962) learning from experience. Class sizes tend to be small, fewer than 20 people, and there is an expectation of 'to and fro', of dialogue and debate. While within theory seminars the seminar leader may begin by explaining certain key points made in a paper set for the seminar and may link it with some ideas, contrast it with others, it is most likely that the participants will also be expected to share their thoughts, bring questions about statements that didn't make sense to them or describe some live clinical experiences which illustrate the concepts. The teaching of clinical skills tends to follow the pattern of a trainee bringing a clinical dilemma or some case material for a smaller group to discuss together. Within the Independent training every week of term there are small group seminars mixed across the year groups, as well as clinical seminars which are held only with those from that year group. From this model we hope to let trainees learn from those at different stages of training, widen their experience of others' thoughts and at the same time recognise the trust that can be built up over time by sharing clinical thinking both within and outside their year group. These seminars invite the trainees to present material – that is, to give a brief anonymised background to the case (occasionally some seminar leaders prefer not to do this and to allow the detailed material to speak for itself) and then to give details of what happened in the room with the specified patient in the course of one meeting. Looking at things in such minute detail, as will be apparent from other chapters in this book, is very much the hallmark of trainings in the psychoanalytically informed tradition (Sternberg 2005).

Supervision as a cornerstone

Child psychotherapy trainees will access supervision in many forms throughout their training. Because in many ways the training is an apprenticeship model, with trainees learning how to be a qualified child psychotherapist by working alongside others, gradually gaining more confidence and autonomy, trainees will be in a placement in a Child and Adolescent Mental Health (CAMH) service, or a voluntary sector organisation offering therapeutic help to children and families, over the four years of their training. In that setting they will be guided by a senior member of the profession who is referred to as a service supervisor. It is part of the condition of the placement that service supervision, of approximately an hour, takes place weekly. It would be expected that during those meetings the trainee talks in detail about their current case load, as well as wider issues, and those needed by line management structures. Some colleagues have pointed out that the 'apprenticeship model' suggests that the experienced colleague has all their abilities at their dexterous fingertips, while the apprentice/trainee has to watch, carefully taking it all in, learning to replicate the craft in a meticulous way. That is certainly not the picture that the idea of an apprenticeship, or at least the journey of learning to be a psychotherapist, conjures up for me: the apprentice/trainee has much to learn, but will learn best by questioning the choices the 'master' has made, watching of course, but while watching silently learning what not to do as well as what to do.

Our trainees have a massive amount of supervision in their working weeks. The system that has become traditional within child psychotherapy trainings, and is to an extent expected by the professional body, the Association of Child Psychotherapists (ACP), is that intensive training cases, i.e., those that are seen (usually) three times a week over at least a year, are each separately supervised by an experienced clinician who is not part of the service, whereas other clinical work (including but not limited to once weekly work, work with parents, assessments and consultations) is supervised by the service supervisor, or occasionally other members of the multidisciplinary team. Over the course of the four-year training a trainee will be expected to work in this intensive way with three cases, spanning the age range, so that they will also over the course of their training have experience of at least three different intensive case supervisors' ways of thinking. The training school has the responsibility for agreeing who should be the intensive case supervisors, and also offering occasional opportunities for Continuing Professional Development (CPD) to them so that they can feel confident about the quality of their thinking and approach. The Independent training has also in more recent years offered additional opportunities for supervision that are not part of the training day. We had used donated funds to enable trainees to seek additional specialist supervision where requested. If a trainee were seeing a case, perhaps with serious physical illness, eating disorders or harmful sexual activity, where they and their Service Supervisor thought that their learning and the work might be enhanced by consultations with someone with an expertise in that area, we would arrange and financially support a limited number of specialist supervisions. We have also been able, through a grant from the Winnicott Trust, to facilitate supervision with someone trained in the Independent tradition if a trainee were placed with a Service Supervisor who was unfamiliar with that approach and who wanted to experience thinking about certain cases using that lens.

Supervision in the context of a training

All these opportunities for individual and group supervision take place within the context of a training. With that in mind we can see that there will inevitably be aspects that unwittingly encourage anxiety and distrust. Trainees know they are being evaluated, and although we have put in systems that try to show how evaluatory processes work (an idea also propounded by Kernberg 2021), the wish to 'do well' and to be seen to be doing well can come to the fore, and predominate over the wish to learn, to discover through not understanding and making mistakes. Casement (2005) warns that supervision within a training institution may not always be straightforward because of issues of power differentials and compliance:

> It could, potentially, inhibit and impair students' learning and development, throughout their training, to be under a pressure to agree with accepted lines of thinking, and to risk being pathologised if they are too vigorous in challenging either what is being taught or the ways in which things are done in the training.
> (Casement 2005: 1147)

He writes of when the creativity of the student's own thinking and emerging ways of working can be stunted when supervision becomes dogmatic and/or controlling. The supervisee has an 'eye over their shoulder', thinking about the supervisor and how they might view the work presented, and this anxious self-watching can lead to feeling paralysed when with the patient. Something similar may also happen with clinical seminars when the fact that the trainee knows that they will present a certain session in an upcoming seminar disturbs the work within the session. He reminds us that:

> Students' fear of failure is such that many of us know of students who have felt the need to edit their clinical accounts of sessions in order to leave out bits that a supervisor might disapprove of, or who have written up a modified account of some session in order to appear to a supervisor or clinical seminar leader, to be interpreting as they are expected to.
> (Casement 2005: 1145)

Kernberg (2018) also speaks of 'submissive atmosphere' and the problem candidates had 'daring to say something new. At the same time, demonstrating how close it was to Freud's thinking' (p. 799).

Within the training day there are further opportunities for supervision taking place in small groups rather than individually, both in practice groups where the trainees mix across the year groups, and in clinical seminars which are in year groups. These are small spaces, where trust develops over time, leading, we hope, to an opportunity to avoid the pitfalls Casement alerts us to and share thoughts freely. The seminar leader is not quite 'one among equals' as there is an acknowledgement of a level of experience, but within the time spent together the seminar leader needs to ensure that everyone is given an opportunity to speak and to have what they say listened to respectfully, and to be open to the trainees coming up with ideas that had not occurred to the seminar leader.

Although it is understood that the trainee presenting the material is the person in the room who knows the patient best, all those present are encouraged to have their own thoughts and to feel free to express them. Some responses may be dominated by emotion, and such strong feelings can also be explored to see whether they may give fresh insights into the case. Throughout training in psychoanalytic psychotherapy from infant observation onwards (Sternberg 2005) observers/trainees/ qualified clinicians are encouraged to approach learning not as accessing 'out there' facts, but as experiences which engage subjective and affective processes. Urwin (2012) writes of infant observation: " Infant observation research generates knowledge not by the collation of facts but by opening new doors and possibilities, inviting readers, via their engagement, to participate in this process" (Urwin 2012: 102).

Gabbard and Ogden (2009) suggest that when confronted with 'novel, disturbing analytic situations' the analyst (whether trainee or qualified) requires another person to 'help make the unthinkable thinkable'. They say, 'That other person is most often the patient, but may be a supervisor, colleague, mentor, consultation group, and so on' (Gabbard and Ogden 2009: 312). Although it can of course at times be a struggle to bear to think differently, it is also essential that an atmosphere of genuine curiosity is encouraged. In an interesting chapter about supervision within a Mentalisation-Based Therapy (MBT)-A context, which states many things which are relevant for supervision within a psychoanalytic framework, Dwyer Hall and Wiwe (2021) state that through 'maintaining curiosity, avoiding labelling, continuously keeping in mind that the less you label and categorise the adolescent the more you recognise that you do not know everything about the adolescent' (Dwyer Hall and Wiwe 2021: 97).

There is – or should be – an atmosphere of 'not knowing'. Surprise – finding out what one does not already know, or indeed finding out that what one thought one knew was incorrect – has long been acknowledged as a central part of learning. In 1646 in his *Pseudodoxia Epidemica* ('common errors') Sir Thomas Browne states 'knowledge is made by oblivion, and to purchase a clear and warrantable body of Truth, we must forget and part with much we know'. He debunks the previously popularly held ideas that 'Children would naturally speak Hebrew' and that 'a Badger hath the Legs of one side shorter than the other'. Indeed! But how did he come to find the falsity of these ideas? I would assume that he did so through looking properly at what was before him. When looking closely again at a session they have been involved in or explaining a family constellation they thought they had understood, through the questions and comments of the seminar group, trainees may discover all sorts of things they did not know or assumptions they had made.

Berman (2000) suggests that the supervisor, and by extension the supervision group, can be an 'invaluable partner' in thinking about the accuracy of patient's attributions to the therapist. Try as we might, we cannot always bear to recognise that, as Searles pointed out as long ago as 1965, what our patients show us they experience us as may not be totally transference based. So, at times the therapist may not recognise that the haughty, self-opinionated other being shown in the play is a version of themselves, or may be comfortable with being seen as the wicked witch because of the transference, but not recognise the ways in which their own ways of being with the patient had engendered this. It is not unusual for different participants to hold identifications with different members of the family or different parts of the network, indeed disentangling these can be a very helpful part and a way in which a group supervision can have advantages over individual supervision. Additional advantages come from the already recognised aspects of group learning such as being able to hear about situations which can be remembered and drawn on in future clinical encounters and becoming aware of other approaches and ways of thinking about issues.

It is important that the training institution and the seminar leaders create an atmosphere in which not having seen something previously, or having made an interpretation that, for example, put the young person into a dysregulated state, can be accepted and looked at as something interesting, not something to be avoided. Slavin addresses how all too often there can be 'adherence to an unwritten set of rules' about how to conduct ourselves with our patients and he thinks of this as often operating out of a 'brittle defensiveness regarding exposure to our patients, and a profound need to guard and control our way of thinking and working' (Slavin 1997: 807).

Berman states: 'A major source of difficulty for supervisees, for example, is that the learning of new skills requires acknowledgement of their lack and such an acknowledgement arouses shame.' When things are going wrong there is the possibility of both supervisor and supervisee experiencing the other as 'threatening judges of each other, both being a potential source of embarrassing exposure and rejection' (Berman 2000: 277). There is a delicate balance that needs to be achieved between being encouraging enough, creating an atmosphere of safety, while still fostering a learning experience in which criticism and concern can be expressed. Within a four-year training it is useful to bear in mind that there will be time for even the most talented trainee to enhance their skills, and certainly time for the ones who have a way to go to indeed develop into fine clinicians. Of course, where the supervisor or seminar leader has strong doubts about the trainee's work this will need to be shared, both directly with the trainee (privately, away from the group if we are thinking about a seminar leader) and with those responsible for the trainee's progress in training. Where there are concerns about the safety of the work, and possible concerns about the welfare of the patient, it is of course important for the seminar leader/supervisor to keep ethical issues in mind, and ensure that those concerns are heard by those in the clinic setting who are responsible for the case.

Helen Morgan makes it clear that:

> In all supervisory relationships the conscious and unconscious dynamics concerning exposure, shame, judgement etc will be present to a greater or lesser extent. Power differentials will exist especially when the supervision is set within a training whereby the supervisor's view will substantially impact on the supervisee's career.

(Morgan 2021: 119)

In *The Work of Whiteness*, she emphasises:

> When differences in race and colour exist within the triad of supervisor, super-
> visee and patient, then an additional layer enters the relationship. This layer will
> include the unconscious dynamics of power, guilt, shame, envy and fear. Being
> irrational and unwanted, these are often difficult matters to think about and dis-
> cuss and, consequently, they are often disavowed.
>
> (Morgan 2021: 119)

Psychotherapists often work with children from families whose culture is alien, or
at least unfamiliar, to them and it is necessary to pay attention to where prejudice
(from both supervisor and therapist) may be impacting on the work. With those
trainees who are people of colour the supervisor and seminar group need also to be
brave enough to mention if they feel that the patient or their family are acting in a
disrespectful way – but first they have to be able to notice it!

A document put out by the ACP in November 2021 collates experiences that
have been discussed by its members and notes, inter alia, the following concerns
related to training. They reiterate that it is important to keep in mind the child's
ethnicity when discussing the case and emphasised how often it can feel as if doing
so becomes the responsibility of those members of the group who are people of
colour, as it may simply not occur to the others. It may be difficult to be the only
black/brown member in a supervision group with a white supervisor, training
schools need to be aware of this and what it might be like.

Particular issues engendered by the pandemic

From Spring 2020 Britain, along with most other parts of the world, was struck
by the Covid-19 pandemic. This tragedy for so many people's lives had an impact
on the work child psychotherapists could do, and on the training, in terms of the
major disruption to trainees' experiences and the delivery of the teaching day. The
teaching day rapidly moved online, and both staff and trainees quickly became
accustomed to making the best of what was available. However, the issue of how
to 'read the room' and how to know when the other is eager to speak caused some
difficulties: the hand up function, together with unmuting, slows down spontaneity. This issue certainly impacted on teaching the seminars in which the emotional responses of the trainees was central. As a seminar leader I have become
accustomed to both hearing clinical material and picking up how that material
is being felt by others. This became more difficult to do. Quieter members, who
perhaps could have been drawn out more in person, could become even quieter,
and invitations to them to share their thoughts could be more easily experienced as
persecutory. One of our teachers described her teaching style as having 'become
like a game show host'.

All of us as clinicians had to discover for ourselves where we wanted to position
ourselves on a spectrum, having regard for the measures that had to be taken to

follow regulations and stay on the safe side, on the one hand, while maintaining the continuity of analyses on the other. Trainees, unlike those in private practice, had to work within the strictures that their management decreed. Sometimes we heard heart-breaking stories of management deciding to 'traffic light' the cases and to close immediately, without further opportunities for saying goodbye, any that did not light 'red' in terms of urgent need. Frequently, because we did not yet understand the virus and how it spread, we heard of children's toys being removed and destroyed. Now the idea of them as 'plague carriers' might seem absurd, and even representing something untamed about disturbed children that had to be got rid of, but at the time we were all bewildered, distressed and certainly feeling impotent. Supervision sessions were filled with reports of weeks and even months going by in which plans for systems to be used were delayed and no contact was made between clinician and patient because it was always hoped that tomorrow would bring resolution. Understandably trainees and other clinicians were not allowed to make contact with their patients except using work-provided phones or laptops, but then the necessary equipment took time to arrive. Child psychotherapists in general, and trainees in particular, were faced with the question of what it was possible to offer and to whom. Even when the family circumstances made connection possible, could a young child have an individual session or would it be necessary to have an adult in the room, turning the work into some sort of parent-child therapy? As one of our intensive case supervisors put it in her end-of-year-report, 'How do you frame comments, observations, interpretations when carer and child are both in the room? Is it carer-child work or carer facilitating the child's individual therapy?' If the child was, as so many of our patients are, dysregulated and acting out, was it safe, even with a slightly older child, to offer individual work which meant that they were in a room alone with the phone or laptop? What to do with the child who was alone and then did physically reckless things? Yet even in services that were very quickly offering in-person work for the most needy children and families, seeing (rightly in my opinion) these as essential medical services, these more 'all over the place' children could not be seen either – their tendency to use their bodies to express their anxieties, their inability to keep distance and not intrude meant they could not be welcomed into these new fragile-feeling clinics, where fear pervaded contact between people.

I want to emphasise what splendid creative work was done in these adverse circumstances. The determination of the trainees to continue to offer some sort of therapeutic contact to the families was admirable. I am surprised and gratified by how much good work the trainees were able to do online. Most of those I supervised used online contact, although some working with adolescent patients or parents used the phone. Those clinicians in services which allowed them to do in-person work were then faced with some of the problems that things were not the same. Clinicians had to wear masks – and early on plastic aprons and gloves too; there was a limitation on the toys available (shared toys were no longer acceptable, the previous box had often been destroyed); often reconfiguration of clinic space meant that the familiar therapy room could no longer be used. Clinics became far less welcoming places, with no use of the waiting room in some services, creating management problems. Some children are still having what I, adapting the term 'blended learning', call 'blended therapy', with not all of their sessions in person, or in a few instances sessions in different physical places, to help with issues of transport or clinic restrictions on room use. From my position as supervisor, it seems that when this model is used there is less sense of continuity between sessions. For those of us who have grown up thinking about the importance of the frame, what does this do to the frame (Langs 1973)? Is it the best compromise or are we so eager to have something ('something is better than nothing') that we have lost sight of what is essential? One of the problems we have seen as a result of the pandemic is that we cannot rely on things continuing as they are. We have already experienced the on/off nature of lockdowns and release and have to keep in mind that the experience of in-person work may now have to be withdrawn – and possibly withdrawn suddenly – before long. Again, in this unknown territory is it better to start something, even if it has to be stopped? Certainly, many therapists and patients think so.

The sense of not knowing what one is doing has also been pervasive for those supervising others during these difficult times. We have been accustomed in our supervisory roles to being able to draw on our own experience. Of course, some of us have not been trainees for many years and even without the pandemic the services we worked in and the patients we saw may bear little resemblance to what today's trainees are having to contend with. But there would be ways of thinking about children, their experiences and the symbolic meaning of their communications that could feel familiar, set against the certainty of certain psychoanalytic ways of understanding. For the 1st 2 years when Covid 19 was most virulent we were in totally uncharted territory. Sebastian Kohon has written an interesting article about this. He writes: 'In our roles as clinicians, supervisors and supervisees, how do we draw on a sense of legitimate authority when, to some extent at least, no-one knows what they are doing?' (Kohon 2020: 281).

The ACP created a number of groups of those supervising to think together about their experiences, and many of us have found them supportive in a number of ways. The group I was in shared its experience of feeling at sea and often used the space for talking about what Kohon terms 'universal existential anxieties brought up by the pandemic (albeit in different manifestations and to differing degrees)' which 'have coincided with sudden changes to the setting'. He draws attention to the fact that 'our supervisors and analysts, whether in reality or as internalised figures, are also in the same frightening and confusing situation. Their functioning, or at least the use we can make of them, may thus be compromised' (Kohon 2020: 286). He raises this interesting idea that under normal circumstances we attribute qualities of wisdom, and perhaps omniscience, to our supervisors and that the inevitable recognition that they/we too are flailing about in the dark may feel disturbing.

As supervisors, we are trying to help supervisees think through clinical dilemmas which are arising in situations that are completely new to everyone. This cannot help but bring us face to face with our own limitations. Recognising that all through one's professional and personal life we will have to open ourselves to new and strange experiences is part of what makes this such a fascinating profession to which to belong. Such acknowledgement of the lack of omniscience – and possibly even lack of wisdom – is actually no bad thing. Berman (2000) writes of the idealisation that teachers and supervisors often receive, and sometimes foster because of their own narcissism. A trainee recognising that teachers and supervisors do not belong to a different order of being, think and act in a way that would forever be out of reach of the trainee, is an important part of learning to be a qualified clinician. Gabbard and Ogden say that the supervisor's awareness and acknowledgement of their own limitations can help shape the trainee to increase their 'humility, curiosity' about themselves, recognising that development and self-understanding are a 'lifelong task' (Gabbard and Ogden 2009: 318).

I have been talking from my perspective as an intensive case supervisor, but of course much of the trainees' learning comes from their non-intensive cases and other pieces of clinical work, usually supervised by the service supervisor. On the whole such supervisions have taken place, but the informal consultation with colleagues, the mopping up that can take place in the kitchen following a distressing session or the support that can be found by popping your head round the door to ask for advice has been sorely missed. One needs to be in a different state to feel free to make a phone call to the supervisor at such times.

Conclusion

When bringing work to a practice group or clinical seminar the presenter should genuinely want to think about the case rather than simply be taking their turn in a rota, and the seminar leader and other trainees should not be using this as an opportunity to show their own clinical skills, finding ways that they might have done better. The importance of this as a learning experience for all involved is crucial. Dwyer Hall and Wiwe (2021) outline a model in which participants actively and quite specifically seek out the problems they are facing to avoid the supervision operating without direction. Yet, as we have noted, the trainee may feel exposed within the setting and want to avoid risk. As much as possible the seminar leader needs to convey that at any time our understanding of what is going on within a treatment is always tentative. Slavin says:

> teaching and supervision has to come from a position of learning together, just as we might expect it to happen in treatment. If it is from the position of the teacher as one who knows and the students as those that do not know, can we expect our candidates to be students with their patients? ... supervisors and teachers will need to approach their task from the same collaborative and vulnerable position that ... we hope our candidates will approach the treatment process.
>
> (Slavin 1997: 816)

Of course, the reader will have noticed those 'shoulds'. Sometimes dynamics within a group lead to something very different. Within the trainee's year group there will naturally be rivalries and different approaches that lead to a jockeying for position or a lack of respect. The seminar leader may need to work hard at times to create an atmosphere in which all those present feel able to contribute and can expect their contributions to be valued. Group dynamics can also be addressed in other parts of the learning experience, with external facilitators being invited.

Within the training school context supervision may at times be experienced as a burden, another task to be managed, or in a way similar to an assignment that needs to be passed rather than learned from, but if the sense of learning and growing can be kept sufficiently in mind we hope it can feel like a great privilege to have what Dwyer Hall and Wiwe refer to as 'another mind to think with' (Dwyer Hall and Wiwe 2021: 90).

Note

This chapter is a version of a paper presented at the Anna Freud National Centre for Children and Families Colloquium in November 2021.

References

Berman, E (2000) Psychoanalytic supervision: the intersubjective development. *International Journal of Psychoanalysis 81*: 273–290.

Bion, W (1962) *Learning from Experience* London: Heinemann.

Browne, T (1646) *Pseudodoxia epidemica: Or, Enquiries into Very Many Received Tenents* London: T H For Edward Dod.

Casement, P (2005) The Emperor's clothes: some serious problems in psychoanalytic training. *International Journal of Psychoanalysis 86* (*4*):1143–1160.

Dwyer Hall, H and Wiwe, M (2021) Varifocal vision in a world of storm and stress. Supervising MBT-A practice. In T Rossouw, M Wiwe and I Vrouva (eds.) *Mentalization-Based Treatment for Adolescents. A Practical Treatment Guide* Hove: Routledge.

Gabbard, G and Ogden, T (2009) On becoming a psychoanalyst. *International Journal of Psychoanalysis 90* (*2*): 311–327.

Kernberg, O F (1986) Institutional problems of psychoanalytic education. *Journal of the American Psychoanalytic Association 34*: 799–834.

Kernberg, O F (2018) Otto Kernberg on 'Institutional problems with psychoanalytic education'. An interview with Otto Kernberg. PEP/CL Top Authors Project.

Kernberg, O F (2021) Challenges for the future of psychoanalysis. *The American Journal of Psychoanalysis 81* (*3*): 281–300.

Kohon, S (2020). Challenges to making use of countertransference responses during the Covid-19 pandemic – some preliminary thoughts. *Journal of Child Psychotherapy 46* (*3*): 283–288.

Langs, R (1973) *The Technique of Psychoanalytic Psychotherapy* Volume *1* New York: Jason Aronson.

Morgan, H (2021) *The Work of Whiteness* Hove and New York: Routledge.

Searles H F (1965) The effort to drive the other person crazy – an element in the aetiology and psychotherapy of schizophrenia. In *Collected Papers on Schizophrenia Related Subjects* London: Karnac.

Slavin, R (1997) Models of learning and psychoanalytic traditions. Can reforms be sustained in psychoanalytic trainings? *Psychoanalytic Dialogues 7* (6): 803–817.

Sternberg, J (2005) *Infant Observation at the Heart of Training* Hove and New York: Routledge.

Urwin, C (2012) Using surprise in observing cultural experiences. In C Urwin and J Sternberg (eds.) *Infant Observation and Research: Emotional Processes in Everyday Lives*. Hove and New York: Routledge.

Chapter 3

Feel the force

The experience of a supervisee on the child and adolescent psychoanalytic psychotherapy training

Ben Yeo

> when we feel the force of our counter-transference, when our own feelings become hard to manage – feelings of being overwhelmed or paralysed, of great sympathy and compassion, or of rage and an internal urge to be angry with the patient or to retaliate sadistically. Space for thinking is vital.
>
> (Horne 2006: 226)

Introduction

In the film *The Empire Strikes Back* (1980), Luke Skywalker pilots his spaceship away from the main action towards a mysterious planet called Dagobah. There, Luke finds a Jedi Master called Yoda who provides the time, space and thinking which help him in his training to become a Jedi. Yoda uses a phrase which echoes the opening quote of the chapter: 'you must feel the force around you, here between you, me … everywhere'. Luke says later, 'I can help them, I feel the force.' During his training, Luke wavers between feelings of excitement, awe, fear and despondency. These emotions relate to the main events of the film but they are also stirred up by Luke's training with Yoda which could be seen as a supervisory encounter. The interactions between Luke and Yoda have been etched on my mind since childhood. More recently, and inspired by the *Star Wars* themed play of my first young training patient, these scenes have also helped me reflect on my experience of being a supervisee on the child and adolescent psychoanalytic psychotherapy training.

The mystery of Dagobah captures my experience of starting the clinical training which at times felt like stepping into an alien world. Before my supervisors take offence, I am not likening any one of them to the wizened 800-year-old Jedi Master. Nor am I admitting to my own grandiose fantasies of being Luke Skywalker. Rather, the scenes between these two characters have helped me to consider the forceful dynamics of supervision. Ogden writes about the 'multiplicity of emotional forces at work in the supervisory relationship' (2005: 1266). This chapter explores the different ways in which I experienced these forces. Supervision offered me a safe and protective space that helped me to 'feel the force' (Horne 2006: 226) of counter-transference feelings for the first time. When these dynamics were explored in

DOI: 10.4324/9781003297604-5

supervision, powerful feelings were stirred up in me towards my supervisors. At times, the same 'emotional storm' (Bion [1979]1987) between me and my patient felt alive in the supervision itself. Learning of any kind can stir up strong emotions and as a supervisee I experienced the combination of 'wondrous excitement and anxious dread' that Wittenberg (1983: 3) suggests is central to the beginning of any learning experience.

A prominent feature of Luke's training is how he learns to develop his vision and to make sense of what he sees. On Dagobah, Luke is helped by Yoda to understand disturbing visions, including one which reveals the true identity of his father – the infamous Darth Vader. The theme of looking is linked to another central idea of this chapter; supervision helped to develop my therapeutic sight in a number of ways, including honing my observation skills and enabling me to hold onto the multiple, and often conflicting, perspectives of my patients.

This chapter charts a personal journey through three supervisory relationships which were central to my clinical training. The identifying features of the patients have been changed and anonymised where appropriate. My hope is that parts of this journey resonate with other supervisees, and could be a helpful reminder for supervisors and training schools of the daunting and exciting experience of being supervised for the first time. Rustin suggests that the role of clinical supervision in the training of child psychotherapists has received 'rather scant attention in the literature' (Rustin 1998: 433). The perspective of the supervisee is one even less represented and I am delighted there is an opening for it in this book.

Supervision one: dragged from a swamp

When Luke enters the skies of Dagobah he is battle-weary and injured. In previous scenes he has narrowly avoided being eaten alive by a wild animal and has fought his way off a planet under attack. Luke loses control of his ship and crash lands into a swamp. The crash landing is an appropriate metaphor for how a supervisee can enter the supervisory relationship, particularly their first one. Rustin captures the experience of being a fledgling trainee:

> intense shock is often experienced by trainees when they encounter the child's capacity for cruelty, self-destructiveness, and perversion and the failure of families and the wider social world to protect children adequately.
>
> (Rustin 1999: 140)

I was disturbed by early clinical encounters with my first training case, a three-year-old adopted boy. He had experienced trauma, neglect and life-threatening injuries from physical abuse in his earliest weeks. My patient's anxiety and concomitant need for control in the treatment room was wearing me down. I struggled to think and felt deskilled, exhausted and physically injured from kicks to the shin. The combination of my lack of clinical experience and the projections of my patient's early fears for survival created a sense of precariousness in me.

Attending supervision at this early stage was the equivalent of being dragged from a swamp. Rustin writes about helping her supervisee who was 'flooded by confused emotion' (Rustin 1998: 447). I saw my young patient in a treatment room where there was water, taps and a sink. In the early phase of treatment, I often finished sessions soaked in water or mopping up puddles from the dysregulated water play of my patient. The flooding was a sign of my difficulties in establishing boundaries both in the treatment room and within myself. A critical task of early supervision sessions, alongside my personal analysis, was to help me survive these primitive projections and to establish a sense of emotional safety for both myself and my patient.

A significant memory of early supervision sessions was being offered cups of tea by my supervisor. Cebon (2007) describes being fed apple strudel, coffee and soup from Esther Bick in supervision. Luke is offered soup and a warm fire by Yoda at the beginning of his training. Perhaps the cups of tea served as the equivalent of a maternal feed and helped to calm my distress, something which had particular resonance to the case; I was treating a young patient whose early infantile experiences had been ruptured by his abusive parents. The terror and impossibility for him of latching on to his earliest parental object was alive in the treatment room and I needed sustenance from my supervisor to fortify me. Goren describes how snacks and drinks now form a staple part of psychotherapy sessions for his traumatised adopted patients whom he describes as needing 'a concrete signal of nurture' (Goren 2020: 157). Perhaps I was hungry for this same sense of nurture in the early phase of supervision.

Once extricated from the proverbial swamp, there was a growing possibility for me to think. The slower and more thoughtful rhythm of supervision was a necessary counterpoint to the frenetic tempo of the treatment room. My patient ricocheted around the room like a pinball, jumping across high surfaces from windowsills to sofa top. I broke out in a sweat trying to follow him around the room. I needed supervision to catch my breath. Horne suggests that supervision is a 'time of calm reflection … something that many children do not grant us in the passion of the therapeutic encounter' (Horne 2006: 225).

Supervision helped to contain my anxiety and I began to be able to observe my patient. My supervisor was sparse with her words, listening to the reading of my process notes, often with her eyes closed. I understand now that her stillness may have been a response to my high volume of words and anxieties – her closed eyes an attempt to bring me closer to a state of reverie and connection with my patient. In the treatment room, I had initially wanted to assert myself as a new therapist and rushed to make interpretations in an attempt to wrest back control. While my patient clambered up and over high surfaces, my convoluted explanations as to why he might be high up, and what he might be trying to avoid through climbing, went unheard by him. By contrast, my supervisor listened attentively to me and held a 'birds-eye view' of the treatment (Lanyado 2016: 108).

With my supervisor in mind, I scaled back my words in the treatment room. When I talked it was simple descriptive statements of what my patient was doing: naming his actions, body movements and noticing aloud just how high up he was. These observations began to capture my patient's attention and over time we felt more connected. This connection helped me to see some of the more ordinary and developmentally appropriate capacities of my patient. I had been rather lost in preoccupations of his history of trauma and abuse. I think this is a common experience for trainees starting out with lots of time to read long, and often highly disturbing, case histories which can obscure the patient coming to the treatment in the here and now.

I began to recognise and nurture the healthy aspects of my patient, especially his potency. My observations became more enthusiastic and celebratory; I suggested to him that he was showing me just *how* big and strong he was feeling. Again, this was a way to build a connection. Given his background, my patient would have been starved of 'narcissistic gratification' at key moments in his short life. I responded to his demands to celebrate his potency and in these moments I adopted the admiring parental gaze which is integral to the phallic narcissistic phase (Edgcumbe and Burgner 1975).

At times I needed to get involved in my patient's play and, encouraged in supervision, I let go of my fantasy of a child psychotherapist who sits calmly in his chair whilst delivering wise interpretations. I entered into my patient's elaborate world of *Star Wars* and superheroes with role-play and light-sabre fight sequences. It felt crucial that my patient was able to assert his aggression and potency in these games without fear of retaliation from me. In this way, I came to represent an increasingly safe parental object for my patient compared to the revengeful and abusive 'Darth Vader'-like father whom he had experienced in his earliest weeks.

A two-year intensive psychotherapy treatment gifted me an opportunity for a two-year supervision. There was time for things to unfold in the treatment room and in the supervisory relationship. The initial phase of supervision provided a holding environment while I was learning to do the same for my patient. This involved helping me to experience the 'shock waves' (Lanyado 2016: 111) of working with traumatised children. Having been rescued from the swamp, supervision began to fuel my confidence and imagination. Feeling contained in supervision enabled me to discover how best to respond to my patient; I learned to observe him, follow his play and over time a playful dialogue opened up between us which set the foundations for the treatment. Perhaps like all first intensive training cases, this treatment was a pivotal moment in my training journey, and it feels appropriate for the *Stars Wars* theme to underpin this chapter.

Supervision two: awe and inadequacy

'For 800 years have I trained Jedi,' Yoda tells Luke Skywalker in The Empire Strikes Back (1980). In response to Yoda's 800 years of experience, Luke feels both inspired and inadequate. In response to Yoda's 800 years of experience, Luke feels both inspired and inadequate. Yoda sets Luke the task of moving objects using just 'the force'. Luke manages to move a heavy boulder and then tries to extricate his crashed spaceship from the swamp. Luke fails and declares: "You want the impossible!", then in a climactic moment (accompanied by rousing music), Yoda steps in and uses the force to raise the spaceship. Luke watches with a sense of awe and hopelessness.

I had the privilege of being supervised by vastly experienced child psychotherapists during my training. Perhaps inevitably these meetings stirred up feelings of awe and inadequacy in me. Hopkins reports similar feelings in the early stages of her supervision with Winnicott; she was:

> over-awed when he agreed to see me. My anxiety increased when he fixed a regular appointment at lunch-time and sat listening to me with closed eyes. I felt sure he would have preferred an after-dinner nap.
>
> (Hopkins [1996]/2015: 135)

Cebon (2007) describes similarly terrified feelings climbing the steps to Esther Bick's apartment for her supervisory sessions. These examples relate to highly eminent supervisors with the psychoanalytic equivalent of 800 years of experience. But perhaps there is a truth to this in any supervisory encounter. As well as being a source of containment and creativity, the gulf in clinical experience between supervisee and supervisor can stir up feelings of falling short in the supervisee.

A typical response early on in my training was to defer my capacities to my supervisor whom I was convinced would have done a much better job than me in every regard. Rustin points to the inevitability of the supervisor starting out as a 'critical super ego figure' (Rustin 1998: 433) for the supervisee. Horne evokes 'The Great Child Psychotherapist in the Sky' (Horne 2006: 225) who lurks over the shoulder of psychotherapists and would do everything correctly and calmly by making succinct mutative interpretations.

Another response in me was to reject my supervisor. Supervision put me in contact with my own sense of 'lack' and I found this hard to tolerate and wanted to escape it. Luke resents the expectations placed on him by Yoda and when his ship is repaired he urgently leaves Dagobah, perhaps prematurely. I desperately needed supervision yet at the same time I resented it and felt I did not need it at all. Crick suggests that the state of mind of supervisees in training and the demands they make of their supervisors are 'as contradictory and paradoxical as the demands familiar to the parents of adolescent children' (Crick quoted in Omand 2009: 34). I was fortunate to have supervisors who contained these forceful feelings. Feelings of inadequacy were acknowledged whilst at the same time there was space for me to assert my capacities and strengths.

I will present an example from the early stages of supervision in my second training case, in which I was helped to understand how my feelings of falling short linked to the primitive projections of my patient.

I was feeling apprehensive in the early stages of supervision in my work with a young adolescent patient. I noticed how these feelings were pervasive and were affecting my preparation for supervision itself. I struggled to write process notes, feeling they were short, lacking in depth and quality. Sometimes I dreaded supervision, weighed down by a sense that my work was not good enough.

I felt stuck and paralysed in the treatment room with my patient, and I felt ashamed to be reporting these feelings to my supervisor. Not content with my own sense of inadequacy, I began to project this into my supervisor; I questioned if she could provide me with what I needed.

Testament to the trust in the supervisory relationship, I was able to share the uncomfortable feelings. I admitted to my supervisor that I felt the work I was bringing her was not good enough. She helped me to see a link between these feelings and the primitive projections of my patient. She suggested that I felt like an unwanted and not good-enough supervisee and this echoed my patient who had a fundamental lack of self-worth shaped by their early experiences.

My patient had been born into a house of neglect and abuse. My patient was physically small and had developmental delays which carried into adolescence. Initially, the patient had no idea how to make use of the therapeutic space and felt they had nothing to offer me. A deep sense of inadequacy was projected into me which in turn I brought into my supervision.

I shared with my supervisor an overwhelming feeling of being stuck with a patient I did not want. It was not just the unpalatable nature of the referral which included rather gruesome details of behaviours which were suggestive of an emerging forensic profile, but I also found the experience of being in the treatment room excruciatingly uncomfortable. My supervisor linked these feelings with the patient's infantile experience of feeling unlikeable and unclaimed by a mother preoccupied with drugs and sexual partners. My patient had not been able to latch onto their early parental object, and I was bringing these same difficulties into my supervision.

The links made by my supervisor provided immediate relief for me and, over time, things began to free up in the treatment room. Holding in mind thoughts of my patient as an unwanted baby helped me to tolerate the painful interactions between us. I felt less paralysed, and I was able to make tentative links with my patient's states of mind. My patient responded by beginning to express themselves, drawing simple pictures reminiscent of a young child. The stuck feelings in the treatment room began to loosen, and my patient began to move around the room and explore the surroundings.

I stopped dreading clinical sessions and in turn my patient began to tolerate the therapy. In a parallel process, I began to relax in my supervision sessions, feeling that I had something of value and worth to share with my supervisor. Over time, my patient became a prolific artist in the treatment room and I added a folder to store the increasingly complex and age appropriate drawings. Similarly, I had more confidence in writing my process notes; the notes became fuller and richer, and where there were gaps I became curious about what this was telling me about the communication of my patient.

Supervision three: the dark side of the force

Luke feels disturbed on Dagobah, especially when he learns the true identity of his sadistic and villainous father (the infamous Darth Vader). The darker side of masculinity links to another training case in which sexual and generational boundaries had collapsed; my young patient disclosed sexual abuse by a male family member during the treatment.

Helping to create a safe space for me and my patient was a central task of supervision. Ralph suggests that when working with children who have been sexually abused, 'the expectation for the child is that the abuse will be repeated in the consulting room' (Ralph 2001: 285). This presented particular challenges for me as a male clinician; I was providing therapeutic space for my patient to process the abuse, but I was also being invited to participate in re-enactments of the abuse. I was in the complex position of being someone who had responded to my patient's disclosures and taken action to keep them safe, whilst also taking on the role in the transference of an abuser, and someone for them to abuse.

Supervision helped me to navigate technical dilemmas inside and beyond the treatment room. I would challenge Szecsody's assertion that supervisors 'should refrain from giving support, advice and suggestions' (Szecsody 2014: 2). When an inexperienced clinician meets a highly disturbed patient, I believe this is exactly what is needed. Initially, the treatment was characterised by aggression, destruction and perversion. In supervision we thought practically about pausing or stopping sessions when things felt overwhelming for my patient (or for me), how to respond to my patient's disclosures, if/when to make safeguarding referrals and how to communicate with the family and the wider professional network about the treatment.

I am indebted to my female service supervisor who provided vital supervision in the early stages of the case. When it became an intensive training case, I needed to find a separate supervisory space, and I sought out a male supervisor. There is little written about gender, or indeed other aspects of identity and difference more generally, in supervision. In this case, I felt that I wanted my gender reflected in my supervisor. Having a safe, benevolent and thinking male figure alongside me was important in countering the abusive versions of masculinity which cast their shadow in the treatment room. I was fortunate enough to find a highly experienced male supervisor but I realise that our profession has a long way to go before supervisees from a diverse range of backgrounds are able to see aspects of themselves reflected in their supervisors.

Emanuel, Miller and Rustin (2002) point to the importance in the supervision of sexual abuse cases of helping the therapist to establish and maintain appropriate boundaries. This is particularly relevant for a group of patients for whom 'a fundamental rule has been broken'. The task of the therapist is 'to give the child a taste of a world where important rules are kept, and the task of the supervisor is to support this'. This was pertinent to my case where the patient continually pushed and tested boundaries. For example, I was often asked by my patient to close my eyes in sessions. This could shift from a playful hide and seek to something with a more sexualised undertone. I was helped in supervision to understand the importance of keeping my eyes open; it was crucial that I hold a firm boundary and assert my position as a thinking adult who could see and try to understand what was happening at all times.

One particular boundary that needed shoring up was between the personal and the professional. There was a risk that the disturbing nature of the clinical material could overwhelm me. The play therapist Janet West (1997) writes compellingly about the impact on professionals of working with sexually abused children. On one occasion, during a series of disclosures, my patient had scrawled felt tip over my hands. That evening at home, I remember working hard to scrub off the ink. In my mind, there were associations between the ink and semen following the ejaculation of an abuser. I had to work hard to free myself from these transference feelings and to limit the impact of the treatment on my home life. I drew on the support structures of my clinical training, including personal analysis and supervision to maintain a sense of emotional safety.

It was both the verbal and nonverbal aspects of supervision which helped me. I remember how during the reading of my process note, my supervisor would follow line by line closely, and I observed him making annotations on his copy of the note. At particularly disturbing moments in the recollection of a clinical session, there would be a pause, a glance, a shared intake of breath or sigh. These exchanges felt like punctuation marks of healthy interaction and reciprocity which helped to diffuse the perverse types of communication filling the treatment room. The 'closed-eye' approach of my first supervisor (which had been appropriate for that case) would not have helped me here. I needed more active containment, reality testing and help in tempering the disturbed world of my patient.

The close attention of my supervisor helped me to gather together what felt like fragments of the clinical material. My patient defended themselves against their emotional states by moving manically between activities and fluctuating states of mind. I struggled to keep up and was often left with a pervasive sense of threat. In supervision we worked in a methodical way to reconstruct the events of the treatment room. I was helped to notice patterns in my patient's behaviour and responses, and this allowed me to anticipate events before things spiralled out of control. A parallel process was at work; supervision helped me to feel more emotionally contained and my patient began to feel safer and more able to tolerate their time in the treatment room.

The gradual and hard-fought developments in my patient over the treatment are beyond the scope of this chapter. Here, I want to draw attention to the changing nature of the supervision itself. Initially, my supervisor helped to cushion the shock and disturbance of working with a traumatised patient. As the treatment progressed, the emotions, which my patient had been so heavily defended themselves against, began to break through. These feelings were named and thought about in the safe space of supervision first, and only then was I able to tentatively express and explore them with my patient in the treatment room. In supervision, I began to experience surges of feeling including terror, sadness, loss and the beginnings of hope. In this way, supervision was not only an 'island of contemplation' (Sterba quoted in Lanyado 2016: 110), it was also a space for powerful and uncomfortable emotions. I felt these counter-transference feelings particularly forcefully, perhaps because my patient was feeling them for the first time themselves. Lanyado describes the process of connection and hope after trauma as 'life reasserting itself after a period of bleak interpersonal numbing' (Lanyado 2016: 108).

My patient's increasing capacity to express themselves helped me to see them as an ordinary young child, not just the child who had been sexually abused. These glimmers of health emerged, but as is so familiar in cases of sexual abuse, they were quickly extinguished by a sadistic or perverse act in the treatment room. Supervision helped me to hold onto my patient's ordinary and appropriate ways of relating, ensuring they were not obscured or lost by the ongoing disorder. In this way I was helped to build up the non-abused aspect of my patient's personality (Alvarez 1992) which was crucial for my patient and also for me to maintain my stamina as a therapist.

Supervision in a changing world

Dagobah is a dark planet shrouded in mist and at first Luke struggles to find his way. This resonated with my experience of entering the treatment room for the first time as a clinician. I had previous experience of working with children and young people in other contexts, but I had never worked in a clinic and I had never been called a 'clinician' ... It felt like stepping into a new world. Phone calls from the receptionist telling me that a patient had arrived for their appointment filled me with terror. Supervision, together with the other supporting structures of my training, helped me to navigate these feelings and to build my confidence in seeing patients. Indeed, my supervisors helped to develop my therapeutic sight in a number of ways.

Supervision helped to hone my observational skills, a central component of the pre-clinical studies of a child psychotherapist (which includes a two-year infant observation and a one-year young child observation). Sternberg (2005) writes about the capacities developed through infant observation and the links with the clinical training of child psychotherapists. As a new therapist, I could easily lose sight of my patients in the treatment room, especially under fire. The case studies in this chapter show how another pair of experienced eyes and a thinking mind helped me to hold onto an observational stance. Sometimes this meant literally keeping my eyes open, at other times it involved not rushing to find meaning and scaling back my interpretations. I also learned to observe the feelings being stirred up in myself. Writing about infant observation, Crick refers to this as the 'third position'; supervision helped me to find within my own mind 'a space in which to think about the felt feelings' (quoted in Sternberg 2005: 91).

The disturbing and strong counter-transference feelings stirred up by clinical encounters could leave me with a fragmented view of my patients. Rustin captures this in her description of her supervisee 'looking through a kaleidoscope' (Ruskin

1998: 438). Supervision helped me to gather together these fragments and to form a more integrated view. I learned to notice my patients' ordinary and developmentally appropriate ways of relating, ensuring these were not obscured or lost by the pathology. Reflecting on these glimmers of health and hope in supervision helped them to grow in the treatment room. As I grow in experience as a child psychotherapist, I understand that my role is to be an advocate of health as well as disorder, and the importance of holding onto both perspectives.

The ending of this chapter has prompted me to consider the 'endings' of the supervisory relationships which were so pivotal to my clinical training. The use of apostrophes conveys how, to some extent, it has not felt like a clean break. Not only am I still in contact with my supervisors since qualifying, I have also felt their continued presence at difficult times in the treatment room. After completing his training, Luke continues to 'see' and be advised by Yoda (and other Jedi Knights) in hologram form!

Now a qualified child psychotherapist, and beginning the journey of being a supervisor myself, I am striving to find my own therapeutic and supervisory voice. This voice comes from within me but it is also a synthesis of my previous supervisory relationships and personal analysis. Contemporary factors are significant here too; the pressures of working in the National Health Service make it even harder to hold onto psychoanalytic thinking with increasingly disturbed patients, families and ever-growing case loads. These factors are heightened as I write this during a global pandemic. Now more than ever it feels crucial to be helped, and to help others, to hold onto an observational stance and to see the multiple and conflicting perspectives of patients, families and the fragmented services that we work in.

Acknowledgements

Thank you to my supervisors (those referenced in this chapter, and more) who continue to inspire me. Thank you, also, to Gautami Parekh and Lyndsey Sharp, two fellow graduates from the Independent Psychoanalytic Child and Adolescent Psychotherapy Association (IPCAPA) for their helpful comments on the chapter.

References

Alvarez, A (1992) *Live Company: Psychoanalytic Psychotherapy with Autistic, Borderline, Deprived and Abused Children* London: Routledge.
Bion, W ([1979]1987) Making the best of a bad job. In *Clinical Seminars and Four Papers* Abingdon: Fleetwood Press7.
Cebon, A (2007) Supervision with Esther Bick 1973–1974. *Journal of Child Psychotherapy 33 (2)*: 221–238.
Edgcumbe, R and Burgner, M (1975) The Phallic-Narcissistic Phase – a differentiation between pre-Oedipal and Oedipal aspects of phallic development. *The Psychoanalytic Study of the Child 30*: 161–180.

Emanuel, R, Miller, L and Rustin, M (2002) Supervision of therapy of sexually abused girls. *Clinical Child Psychology and Psychiatry 7* (*4*): 581–594.

Goren, A (2020) 'Something else' in child psychotherapy with traumatised adopted children. *Journal of Child Psychotherapy 46* (*2*):152–167.

Hopkins, J (1996) From baby games to let's pretend. The achievement of playing. In A Horne and M Lanyado (eds.) *An Independent Mind: Collected Papers of Juliet Hopkins* Hove and New York: Routledge, 2015.

Horne, A (2006) Interesting things to say and why. In M Lanyado and A Horne (eds.) *A Question of Technique: Independent Psychoanalytic Approaches with Children and Adolescents* London: Routledge.

Lanyado, M (2016) Transforming despair to hope in the treatment of extreme trauma: a view from the supervisor's chair. *Journal of Child Psychotherapy 42* (*2*): 107–121.

Ogden, T H (2005) On psychoanalytic supervision. *The International Journal of Psychoanalysis 86*: 1265–1280.

Omand, L (2009) *Supervision in Counselling and Psychotherapy: An Introduction.* Basingstoke: Palgrave Macmillan.

Ralph, I (2001) Countertransference, enactment and sexual abuse. *Journal of Child Psychotherapy 27*(*3*): 285–301.

Rustin, M (1998) Observation, understanding and interpretation: the story of a supervision. *Journal of Child Psychotherapy 24* (*3*): 433–448.

Rustin, M (1999) The training of child psychotherapists at the Tavistock Clinic: philosophy and practice. *Psychoanalytic Inquiry 19*:125–141.

Sternberg, J (2005) *Infant Observation at the Heart of Training* London: Karnac.

Szecsody, I (2014) Supervision as a mutual learning experience. In J Savage Scharff (ed.) *Clinical Supervision of Psychoanalytic Psychotherapy* London: Karnac.

The Empire Strikes Back (1980) film director Irvin Kershner, producer Gary Kurtz.

West, J (1997) Caring for ourselves: the impact of working with abused children. *Child Abuse Review 6*: 291–297.

Wittenberg, I S (1983) The emotional aspects of learning. In I S Wittenberg, G Henry and E Osborne (eds.) *The Emotional Experience of Learning and Teaching* London: Karnac.

Chapter 4

Research supervision and its role in the training of child psychotherapists

Evrinomy Avdi

This chapter explores the role of research training and supervision in the professional development of psychoanalytic child psychotherapists. It draws upon my experience of supervising several cohorts of trainees on the Doctorate in Independent Child and Adolescent Psychotherapy, provided by IPCAPA in collaboration with the Anna Freud Centre, as well as trainees' own written accounts regarding their experience. In recent years, there have been several debates concerning psychoanalytic training (Auchincloss and Michels 2003; Kernberg 2016), as well as the role of research in psychotherapy training more generally (McLeod 2013) and in the training of psychoanalytic child psychotherapists more specifically (Fonagy 2009; Rustin 2009). These debates are beyond the scope of this chapter but provide an important backdrop to the issues – strengths, tensions and obstacles – associated with a psychoanalytic clinical training integrated with doctoral-level research. In order to complete the professional doctorate, trainees spend four years on clinical placements in National Health Service (NHS) Child and Adolescent Mental Health Services, where they gain clinical experience in providing both intensive and non-intensive psychoanalytic psychotherapy under supervision, attend theoretical seminars and have personal analysis. During this time, they also conduct a literature review and an empirical study on a topic related to child psychotherapy and write a reflective commentary on their experience of training. For the purposes of this chapter, the reflective commentaries of 11 completed doctoral theses were examined; the key themes relating to the trainees' experience of research were identified and these are discussed in the sections that follow.

Clinical and research supervision: parallel processes?

Several studies have shown that hands-on experience with clients, supervision and personal therapy are the most important factors in the professional development of therapists across the career span (Hill and Knox 2013; Orlinsky, Botermans and Rønnestad. 2001). Clinical supervision aims to help trainee therapists become competent clinicians and plays a key role in the development of their self-efficacy, self-awareness, skill acquisition, clinical expertise

DOI: 10.4324/9781003297604-6

and competence (Hill *et al.* 2017; McWilliams 2021). Supervision is also central to the development of therapist identity (Skovholt and Rønnestad 2003) and there is some evidence that it impacts on client outcomes (Hill et al. 2017). In psychoanalytic trainings, supervision is considered their 'signature pedagogy', i.e., the primary form of teaching through which therapeutic competence is built, as theoretical knowledge becomes linked with clinical practice (Watkins 2011). Similarly, the aim of doctoral supervision is to help develop students' skills and confidence so that they become independent researchers. In the context of the professional doctorate, this also includes promoting trainees' research literacy and research-mindedness, so that future psychoanalytic child psychotherapists are able to navigate the complex and competing demands of contemporary health service provision, generate new knowledge through research, critically evaluate research evidence, increase self-reflection and provide ethical and effective clinical services.

Doctoral supervision has been described as entailing two complementary dimensions, namely, technical and social support, and the combination of these defines different supervisory styles (Lee 2007; Moxham, Dwyer and Reid-Searl 2013). Some research supervisors perceive their role as providing primarily guidance regarding methodological and conceptual aspects of research, whereas others focus on providing social and emotional support. It is generally agreed, however, that supervisors need to be able to assess students' changing needs as they progress through their doctoral studies and adapt their supervisory style accordingly (Lee 2008). Despite individual differences, many students require more direction, guidance and structure in supervision in the early stages and prefer a more hands-off approach as they advance through their studies. For supervisors, this developmental trajectory often translates into striking a balance between support and challenge, in the attempt to foster reflection and critical thinking so that the student gradually 'finds their voice' as a researcher. Several authors draw upon concepts from developmental theory, such as Vygotsky's 'zone of proximal development' and scaffolding, to conceptualise the role of tolerable anxiety in promoting learning.[1] Much of the research supervisor's work entails helping trainees manage the anxiety and frustration that is common in doctoral studies. This parallels clinical supervision, where the creation of a 'holding environment' (Winnicott 1960) is paramount, especially for novice therapists. Supervisors – research and clinical – may initially assume more of a teaching role, which is gradually reduced as the trainee gains experience and confidence (Rønnestad et al. 2018). Mostly, however, the supervisor's task is to provide a reflective space characterised by 'liberating containment', a safe, non-shaming place where supervisees can expose their work and reflect upon it (Ogden 2005; Watkins 2014). Reflection requires tolerance of ambiguity and uncertainty, capacity for cognitive complexity, metacognition (i.e., thinking about thinking), openness to experience, the ability to process negative affect, as well as openness to alternative approaches and methods (Rønnestad and Skovholt 2013) and, as such, is an emotionally demanding position to achieve.

In the professional doctorate, training in research takes place alongside clinical training, and it is crucial to take this context into account when considering the role of research supervision in the developing professional identity of psychoanalytic child psychotherapists. Completing a doctoral thesis relies on several competencies, including the ability to systematically search, synthesise and critically review a broad range of literature; formulate a clinically relevant and appropriate research question; develop and master the conceptual and methodological skills systematically to investigate the research question; make sense of findings within the framework of psychoanalytic theoretical and clinical literature, and communicate these findings in an academic and clinically relevant manner. Trainees are expected to develop these research competencies alongside an intensive and demanding clinical training. Forging an analytic identity is a long, challenging, often painful and sometimes demoralising process (Gabbard and Ogden 2009; Watkins 2014) and the emotional, intellectual and time demands of training must not be underestimated. In addition to time constraints, which limit the opportunities for trainees to immerse themselves in their research and thus allow their project to develop organically, there are several other obstacles to engagement in research, both personal and institutional; these are discussed in the following sections and are conceptualised in the context of the trainees' developmental trajectory.

The central role of the supervisory relationship

In the context of doctoral studies, the relationship the student has with their supervisor has been shown to be a key factor affecting thesis completion (Moxham et al. 2013). Moreover, the quality and amount of research supervision play an important role in students' overall doctoral experience (Pyhältö, Vakalaand Keskinen 2015). Difficulties in the supervisory relationship or inadequate supervision are considered the most significant obstacles to timely thesis completion (Lee 2008), an important consideration given that the rates of withdrawal from doctoral research are generally high (Litalien and Guay 2015).

The apprentice-master model has been dominant in the literature on research supervision. Increasingly, however, supervision is conceptualised as a collaborative venture, entailing a broad range of different learning experiences that are significantly affected by the nature of the supervisor-supervisee relationship (Benmore 2014). A key concept in clinical supervision is the *learning* or *supervisory alliance*. In line with models of the therapeutic alliance, the supervisory alliance is seen to comprise three interrelated components: rapport and a positive emotional bond, collaboratively reached goals and collaboratively agreed tasks (Bordin 1983; Watkins 2014). Although the term is not widely used in the literature on research supervision, its key elements are recognised as crucial for the students' progress. Discrepancies in the expectations of supervisors and students regarding their respective roles and responsibilities have been shown to have a negative impact on the supervisory alliance and open discussions regarding expectations about supervision as well as supervisory 'contracts' have been recommended as ways to avoid such difficulties (Lee 2008; Moxham et al. 2013).

Managing expectations regarding supervision, however, is arguably more complex in the context of the professional doctorate, given that trainees are exposed to different supervisors for the various components of the training. Compared to clinical supervision, research supervision is less regular, takes place in a group format and there is an expectation for trainees to work fairly independently from the start. In their reflective commentaries, several trainees noted their difficulty in navigating different supervisory relationships and described their relationship with their research supervisor as less intimate and containing, at least initially. Nevertheless, for many this changed with time, as their research supervisor gradually acquired the characteristics of an internal object that supported their developing researcher identity, especially during challenging times, as illustrated in the extract below.

> In a process that seemed comparable to that experienced by the Mother and Baby, I experienced a change in how I related to my research supervisor. We began to talk more. Her words kept alive the idea that there was a viable research project in examining (… [omitted for anonymity]). In this way, she became a fixed point around which I could organise myself, in the same way that Bick describes how a disintegrated infant will fix on an object outside of themselves to hold themselves together. I had gained enough understanding to be able to use my supervisor as a new developmental object (…) Having said this, however, I still relied heavily upon my supervisor. I unconsciously placed her in a parental-like position which held together a coherent image of a fully integrated post-doctoral researcher to which I could aspire.

In addition to the more conscious, ego-related aspects of the supervisory relationship that are reflected in the concept of the supervisory alliance, unconscious, affectively charged processes, anxieties, defences and identifications are at play when learning to be a psychotherapist (Gabbard and Ogden 2009). In my experience, similar processes take place in learning to do research and these colour trainees' relationship with their supervisor and affect their engagement with research. Some attitudes towards research are arguably associated with infantile states of mind and result from defensive responses against the anxieties associated with learning, the realisation that research is complex and the recognition that learning entails frustration, confusion, bewilderment and anxiety (Salzberger-Wittenberg, Williams and Osborne 1983). The difficulties in tolerating the experience of not-knowing during one's doctoral research are vividly described in the following extract.

> My supervisor advised me to take time over the findings, and even though I was keen to just get on with it, her words were apposite. In a process akin to digestion, I sat with information I had gathered and then discussed the findings and their implications with her. At this time, I drew on the idea of staying with not knowing something that Bion termed negative capability. I was required to tolerate the discomfort and confusion and not resort to my defences. I had to bear

the physical and emotional pain lodged in my mind and body whilst I reflected on my struggle to incorporate the different bits of information I had gathered.

In response to such anxieties, supervisors are sometimes positioned as the source of all knowledge, with an accompanying expectation that knowledge will be imparted with little effort on the trainees' part. A key function of research supervision, however, is to provide a space for reflection and promote independent thinking. Therefore, expectations of quick answers are often frustrated and, as a result, supervisors may be experienced as inadequate, withholding or punitive. Another common dynamic in the student-supervisor relationship relates to the infantile wish to be fully understood, cared for and supported. Although providing support is an important aspect of the supervisory role, this needs to be disentangled from the wish for the supervisor to provide for all the trainee's needs, which would foster passivity and inhibit development. In addition, the evaluative aspect of the research supervisor's role in providing feedback on academic work may be experienced as judging, leading to distress and a sense of inadequacy. Arguably, this is compounded by the fact that most trainees have little or no experience of research when they embark on their training. Several report feeling unskilled and anxious about research and many actively avoided engaging in research prior to training. The destabilisation that many novice therapists experience when they embark on clinical work may further exacerbate anxieties about being judged and a sense of inadequacy (Orlinsky, Botermans and Rønnestad 2001).

Given the above, the negative potential of supervision must not be underestimated; the power differential and vulnerability of the supervisee in relation to their supervisor, the evaluative function of supervision and, in some cases, lack of supervisor competence are all factors that can contribute to negative supervision experiences. In clinical work, several possible negative aspects of clinical supervision have been reported, including conflicts, restricted or distorted communication, lack of openness and impasses (McWilliams 2021). Such experiences can be intensely disruptive, lowering trainees' self-confidence and trust in themselves, and may evoke negative counter-transference reactions towards clients (Rønnestad et al. 2018). Similar processes can take place in the context of research supervision and, therefore, it is important for research supervisors to be nonjudgmental, emotionally intelligent and flexible, so as to adapt to students' needs (Lee 2007).

The emotional experience of engaging in research whilst training

Several large-scale, international studies on the professional development of psychotherapists of different theoretical orientations and levels of experience have shown that the period of training is characterised by intense anxiety (Rønnestad et al. 2018). In addition to the anticipation, excitement and aspirations associated with new learning, many trainees embark on their training with feelings of anxiety and fear of failure; many come to feel overwhelmed in their role, experience anxiety about their performance and doubt their ability to meet required standards, whilst some assume a position of 'true believer' (Gabbard and Ogden 2009; Orlinsky et al. 2001).

It is widely recognised that trainees are faced with varied and emotionally intense experiences, primarily related to their encounters with clients and novel clinical situations, and many novice therapists are surprised by the intensity of their emotional responses to clinical work (Skovholt and Rønnestad 2003). As training advances and some of the initial anxieties subside, trainee therapists often become aware of the complexity of clinical work and recognise that the theories they draw on need to be contextualised and adapted to individual needs; this realisation may lead to further destabilisation and confusion. In addition, the sense of competence of novice therapists is often dependent on client improvement and their professional identity is not yet sufficiently solid to tolerate narcissistic wounds. The combination of these factors may result in common clinical experiences – such as not managing to establish a satisfactory therapeutic alliance with clients and high drop-out rates – being particularly distressing to trainees. At the same time, the trajectory of doctoral research is rarely smooth and usually entails false starts and periods of feeling stuck or lost in the process. Arguably, the emotional experience of engaging in research during training is greatly affected by the anxieties and emotional work associated with learning to be a psychotherapist. The key aspects of this experience, as reported in the trainees' reflective commentaries, are discussed below.

Most trainees used metaphors to describe their experience of learning, growth and the challenges they faced along the way. Many used the metaphor of a journey, whilst others drew on psychoanalytic developmental theories, such as Winnicott's theory of maturational processes (Winnicott 1965). For most, the journey was not smooth; they described intense feelings, including helplessness, a sense of inadequacy, frustration, feeling daunted and overwhelmed, ambivalence, as well as excitement and personal growth. When referring to the different elements of their training, many referred to their sense of 'juggling' as they attempted a 'balancing act' and struggled simultaneously to 'learn two languages'. For many, research was initially 'a box to be ticked', a 'necessary evil' in their training. Ambivalence about research and defensive splitting between the research and clinical components of the training featured strongly in most accounts. The following extract evokes the initial disillusionment, disorientation, and lack of interest in research that was often reported.

The language being used felt alien, the surroundings and environment mismatched, and I felt hugely disorientated. I was aware that Anna Freud had accommodated the Wednesday case discussions in the library where we now sat discussing statistics. The Freud statue was looking down at the students, and various books on psychoanalytic history and wisdom were there to be viewed, while statistics were being taught as a part of research methods. It was a strange experience, and I found myself fantasizing about doing a 'proper' psychoanalytic training, with cases being discussed as subjects of research. I had a sad sense that I had come to the training at a time when something very valuable was being lost (...) Although encouraged to see my training all as one interlinked process, I could see my engagement and libido far more invested in the theory seminars and in my clinical practice. (...) My attitude regarding clinical work as the authentic work, and research as something for others, carried on within me in an unconscious way. Consciously, I was so happy to be travelling to London and doing the training.

In retrospect, most trainees interpreted their initial ambivalence as resulting from anxieties relating to starting a demanding training and an associated sense of inadequacy, as well as conflicts around the development of their psychoanalytic identity. Several commented that they managed these anxieties through splitting and projecting all that is unwanted, boring, tedious, burdensome on to research.

Now, from my post-qualification position as a working psychotherapist I realise how all-encompassing my anxiety was in beginning a new training and career (...) The encounter with new ways of thinking stirred primitive insecurities. I felt overwhelmed and one of the ways this found expression was through an adolescent-like resistance to taking in new information. I found expressions like 'boring', and 'what's the point' pop into my head when I struggled with the statistics seminar as I tried to make sense of p-values.

Many managed these anxieties through resistance to engaging with their research project, often expressed through avoiding meeting with their supervisors or progressing with their study. Interestingly, such responses were rarely recognised as signs of resistance but were generally attributed to urgent clinical demands or other training commitments. In such situations, research supervisors may experience frustration and helplessness, possibly as a result of trainees' projections. Other trainees became overly needy, dependent and helpless, disavowing their agency and responsibility for their work. During these times, supervisors often experienced a conflict between providing increased guidance versus the need to foster trainees' autonomy and agency. Some trainees managed their anxiety by devaluing research or rebelling against it, whilst others tried to avoid thinking by rushing to conclusions.

I was faced in supervision by the limits of my own understanding about what would constitute 'good' research, and on several occasions left feeling frustrated that I would need to think again about what I wanted to do. On reflection, I think I was overwhelmed by the task of designing my research, and my way of managing this was to prematurely grasp at ideas that I hoped would give me a feeling of security. When my ideas were challenged in supervision I struggled to know how to respond, as they did not have sufficiently strong foundations to withstand much scrutiny. This was a period of pseudo-maturity in my research journey, and it was painful to discover what I had yet to learn and to slowly allow my project to come together step by step. I was aware that some of my learning in the clinical side of the training was taking a similar trajectory and, on several occasions, I found myself feeling disarmed when my cases evolved in a way that made me question the understanding I had previously held.

Several trainees reported that their resistance to research was maintained, and in some cases encouraged, through their encounters with senior members of the profession. Training involves the gradual development of a new professional identity and this is partly mediated through identification with senior therapists, whom trainees often idealise (Gabbard and Ogden 2009; Kernberg 2016). Several trainees reported their confusion and difficulty, when faced with senior colleagues and supervisors who were indifferent or even hostile to research.

> I fought to remain curious and to find my own identity within what I was understanding to be a changing profession, grappling with issues of loss and identity and perhaps not yet certain of what was to be gained by integrating research skills into a clinical training (…) This left me, as a trainee psychotherapist and fledging researcher, eager to integrate these multiple realities and identities, struggling to find colleagues who I could identify with.

In time, trainees' responses to research shifted, their anxiety and defences decreased and they became curious and reflective about their own responses. They began to experience the clinical and research components of their training as interlinked, integrated and, to a large extent, complementary, as described in the following extracts by two trainees.

> The thoughtful process of getting the level of interpretation just right for IPA[2] interestingly helped me reflect on my clinical practice of interpretation with my patients (…) Furthermore, having been used to reflect on key themes in my clinical practice, the task in doing this in my IPA study did not feel alien or arduous. In fact, it felt very similar to a skill I was attempting to master in the therapy room within a different context and applied in a different way.
>
> The difficulties of data analysis seemed to find parallels in the development of clinical technique, too. I was being trained in the art of psychoanalytic interpretations and practicing the level of sensitivity and depth of them in my clinical cases. Parsons (2009) suggested that there is an art to "waiting" as an analyst. The "waiting analyst" is not one that is doing nothing, but rather attuning to the patient. This skill, like that of the thematic analysis, is developed under careful direction and supervision. (…) Furthermore, in the Independent tradition I was learning reliance on theoretical understanding might prohibit imaginative freedom in the therapy room. This appeared so relevant to conducting data analysis, too.

Many trainees reported that their reading for research broadened their knowledge base, challenged previously held assumptions and made them more open to multiple perspectives, in addition to helping them become more adept at critically reading research literature. Moreover, the majority recognised that their research topic was intimately linked to their clinical experience, and, for many, to their personal history. In time, the difference in perspective introduced by research was experienced as a resource, rather than a difficulty, with several trainees referring to psychoanalytic concepts such as transitional space (Winnicott 1953) or the analytic third (Ogden 2004) to describe the effects of these differing perspectives:

> Overall, my experience of undertaking a research project while being clinically trained followed a gradual trajectory of choices that both consciously and unconsciously matched the clinical experiences I was having. Although this trajectory was not always smooth, I believe that it was through making careful choices that the 'merging' of the two worlds was facilitated. Finally, it was within that new, 'third area', created as a result of this process, that I allowed myself to creatively engage in my research study.

Several trainees drew parallels between their own internal processes whilst engaging with their research and the clinical phenomena they were studying, in a process reminiscent of the concept of parallel process in clinical supervision, discussed earlier.

> As in the statistics seminars I was required to attend, I felt out of my depth and acutely aware of my lack and limitations. On reflection, these early encounters with new systems and new ways of thinking mirrored the fledgling efforts of a young child to construct their identity. Mirroring the experience of an infant's arrival into its family, it was as if I had landed in to pre-existing adult structures and was expected to work out my place and role within them.

In evaluating their training as a whole, the majority of trainees reported gratitude for the opportunity to learn about research and clinical work and recognised that their training in research contributed to the development of their clinical work and professional identity. Many reported a commitment to incorporating research in their future careers, as summed up by these two final extracts.

> My outlook on research has changed a lot through this training. I am more aware of the importance of research in child psychotherapy and it also does not appear to me as something completely separate to clinical practice. (...) The analytic skills and the sense of working with my feelings and intuition was similar to clinical work except for the sense of working under attack. I will not be afraid if future jobs include auditing or researching, in fact I might initiate it myself.
>
>   I approach the end of my training feeling certain that I will continue to be engaged with research throughout the rest of my career (...) I feel that it is the

task of the new generation of CAPs [Child and Adolescent Psychotherapists] whose training has given them this dual research and clinical literacy, to bring these two worlds more closely together so that each can enrich the other.

Concluding reflections

Based on their written accounts, the process of conducting a doctoral level research project as part of clinical training was a demanding process for the majority of trainees. In the beginning stages, most experienced the research and clinical components as separate and many reported strong ambivalence towards research. Gradually, however, all trainees reported that they experienced their clinician and researcher identities becoming more integrated, and they recognised overlap and the potential for mutual enrichment between the different competencies associated with each. In this sense, integration seems to be a developmental achievement rather than the starting point of training for many novice psychoanalytic child psychotherapists. Several factors, including time constraints, anxiety and ambivalence towards research – on personal and institutional levels – seem to have a negative impact on the trainees' curiosity and sense of playfulness that are prerequisites for learning. Research often became the receptacle of projections of all that is burdensome and unwanted in their training journey. A key task of research supervision in this process involves managing trainees' anxieties and ambivalence, as well as guiding them through the conceptual and methodological decisions involved in conducting a research study. The aim is to create a space of curiosity, spontaneity, play and a meaningful engagement with research, so that trainees find their voice as a researcher, while following a rigorous and systematic approach to knowledge.

Notes

1 See Daniels, H. (2017). Introduction to Vygotsky. London: Routledge, for a useful introduction.
2 IPA stands for Interpretative Phenomenological Analysis, a qualitative research method

References

Auchincloss, E L and Michels, R (2003) A reassessment of psychoanalytic education: controversies and changes. *The International Journal of Psychoanalysis 84* (2): 387–403.
Benmore, A (2014) Boundary management in doctoral supervision: how supervisors negotiate roles and role transitions throughout the supervisory journey. *Studies in Higher Education 41* (7): 1251–1264.
Bordin, E S (1983) A working alliance model of supervision. *The Counseling Psychologist 11*: 35–42.
Fonagy, P (2009) Research in child psychotherapy: progress, problems and possibilities? In N Midgley, J Anderson, E Grainger, T Nesic-Vuckovic and C Urwin (eds.) *Child Psychotherapy and Research: New Approaches, Emerging Findings* London: Routledge.
Gabbard, G O and Ogden, T H (2009) On becoming a psychoanalyst. *The International Journal of Psychoanalysis 90* (2): 311–327.

Hill, C E and Knox, S (2013) Training and supervision in psychotherapy: evidence for effective practice. In M J Lambert (ed.) *Bergin and Garfield's Handbook of Psychotherapy and Behavior Change* (sixth edition) New York: Wiley.

Hill, C E, Spiegel, S B, Hoffman, M A, Kivlighan, D M, Jr and Gelso, C J (2017) Therapist expertise in psychotherapy revisited. *The Counseling Psychologist, 45 (1)*: 7–53.

Kernberg, O F (2016) *Psychoanalytic Education at the Crossroads: Reformation, Change and the Future of Psychoanalytic Training* London: Routledge.

Lee, A M (2007) Developing effective supervisors: concepts of research supervision. *South African Journal of Higher Education 21 (4)*: 680–693.

Lee, A M (2008) How are doctoral students supervised? Concepts of doctoral research supervision. *Studies in Higher Education 33 (3)*: 267–281.

Litalien, D and Guay, F (2015) Dropout intentions in PhD studies: a comprehensive model based on interpersonal relationships and motivational resource. *Contemporary Educational Psychology 41*: 218–231.

McLeod, J (2013) *An Introduction to Research in Counselling and Psychotherapy* London: Sage.

McWilliams, N (2021) *Psychoanalytic Supervision* London: Guilford Press.

Moxham, L, Dwyer, T and Reid-Searl, K (2013) Articulating expectations for PhD candidature upon commencement: ensuring supervisor/student 'best fit'. *Journal of Higher Education Policy and Management 35 (4)*: 345–354.

Ogden, T H (2004) The analytic third: implications for psychoanalytic theory and technique. *The Psychoanalytic Quarterly 73 (1)*: 167–195.

Ogden, T H (2005) On psychoanalytic supervision. *The International Journal of Psychoanalysis 86 (5)*: 1265–1280.

Orlinsky, D E, Botermans, J-F and Rønnestad, M H (2001) Towards an empirically grounded model of psychotherapy training: four thousand therapists rate influences on their development. *Australian Psychologist 36 (2)*: 139–148.

Parsons, M (2009) An Independent theory of clinical technique. *Psychoanalytic Dialogues 19*: 221–236.

Pyhältö, K, Vakala, J, and Keskinen, J (2015) Fit matters in the supervisory relationship: doctoral students and supervisors' perceptions about the supervisory activities. *Innovations in Education and Teaching International 52 (1)*: 4–16.

Rønnestad, M H, Orlinsky, D E, Schroder, T A, Skovholt, T M and Willutski, U (2018) The professional development of counsellors and psychotherapists: implications of empirical studies for supervision, training and practice. *Counselling and Psychotherapy Research 19 (3)*: 214–230.

Rønnestad, M H and Skovholt, T M (2013) *The Developing Practitioner: Growth and Stagnation of Therapists and Counselors*. London: Routledge.

Rustin, M (2009) What do child psychotherapists know? In N Midgley, J Anderson, E Grainger, T Nesic-Vuckovic and C Urwin (eds.) *Child Psychotherapy and Research: New Approaches, Emerging Findings* London: Routledge.

Salzberger-Wittenberg, I, Williams, G and Osborne, E (1983) *The Emotional Experience of Learning and Teaching* London: Routledge.

Skovholt, T M and Rønnestad, M H (2003) Struggles of the novice counselor and therapist. *Journal of Career Development 30 (1)*: 45–58.

Watkins, C E (2011) Celebrating psychoanalytic supervision: considering a century of seminal contribution. *Psychoanalytic Review 9 (3)*: 401–418.

Watkins, C E (2014) The supervisory alliance: a half century of theory, practice, and research in critical perspective. *American Journal of Psychotherapy 68 (1)*: 19–55.

Winnicott, D W (1953) Transitional objects and transitional phenomena: a study of the first not-me possession. *The International Journal of Psychoanalysis 34*: 89–97.

Winnicott, D W (1960) The theory of the parent-child relationship. *The International Journal of Psychoanalysis 41*: 585–595.

Winnicott, D W (1965) *The Maturational Processes and the Facilitating Environment* London: Routledge, 2018.

Chapter 5

On service supervision

Martin Daltrop

Introduction

The relationship between being a Child and Adolescent Mental Health Services (CAMHS) clinician and being a child psychotherapist is not always an easy one: the two roles and identities require differing but overlapping skills and experience. Navigating these competing demands can be difficult and entails constant review, in line with ongoing changes to the settings and expectations of the service. Service supervision plays a key part in this process.

The National Health Service (NHS) is a complex organisation which sits at the heart of British consciousness and identity. It is a symbol of British culture and values and a source of national pride and love, exemplified by its place at the centre of the opening display of the 2012 London Olympics and, more recently, the weekly public applause offered to its employees during the Covid pandemic. It is also denigrated when things go wrong, as evidenced by increasing numbers of complaints. Similarly, politicians compete to demonstrate their appreciation of the NHS, while at the same time proposing yet new schemes to control it. The strikes within the NHS that began at the end of 2022 at least in part reflected employees' concerns about the insufficient levels of service.

There are huge pressures on resources in many areas of healthcare, including a significant escalation in demand for treatment within CAMHS. This has created a need for interventions that allow large numbers of children and young people to be assessed, treated and discharged rapidly, so as to stretch services as far as possible. This runs counter to the traditional view of child psychotherapy as a long-term treatment, requiring input for parent and child. In relation to other treatments, child psychotherapy can be perceived as an intensive and uneconomic resource.

Child psychotherapists working in the NHS have had to adapt to these pressures, to offer treatments modified from the 'ideal' taught in training. For example, the idea of open-ended treatments, with regular parallel parent work offered by a separate clinician (preferably psychanalytically informed) is seen as a luxury in services where there is a heavy demand on limited clinical resources. Likewise, it can be unrealistic to expect a case to be managed by a second colleague, who will liaise with schools, social care and other agencies to free the clinician to focus exclusively on the work with the child.

DOI: 10.4324/9781003297604-7

The reality of limited resources has led to more 'applied' work which is not necessarily seen as core to child psychotherapy training – though it is acknowledged and thought about in seminars and discussion groups. Child psychotherapists also take on a broader range of clinical work than was once considered within their remit. Most services will expect clinicians to be involved in processing referrals, screening calls, offering generic assessments, doing clinical triage and risk assessments, making secondary referrals and attending accident and emergency departments to offer crisis assessments. Other requirements might depend on clinical specialties, such as within looked after children's services, which offer specialist consultations, or neurodevelopmental teams, which link to community paediatric services or special schools.

In addition to clinical activities, there are many other aspects to the role of a CAMHS clinician. These include the operational running of the service, contributing to systems for referral and assessment, helping the service adapt to changes in commissioning, strategic planning and contributing to the day-to-day assurance process involving data collection and adherence to clinical and operational standards. As part of helping the service to meet the demands from clients and other stakeholders and the requirements of commissioners, child psychotherapists need continually to reflect on and adapt to their role within the service. This involves ensuring that clinical interventions offered not only reflect the integrity of their discipline but also meet the needs of the service in an ever-changing work environment. In the face of pressure on resources, a relatively labour-intensive and specialist discipline needs to actively demonstrate its relevance and cost-effectiveness, to show that its clinicians are working effectively.

Child psychotherapists will be involved in the local team and wider organisational structures at different levels – from trainee and junior clinical level to senior clinician actively involved in leadership tasks. Jobs therefore involve a combination of familiar psychotherapeutic work and complex hybrids of clinical and organisational activities. Supervision that can explore and make sense of this balance of activities – from understanding challenging clinical material to negotiating the different roles within the organisation – is essential to functioning in these roles. The focus of supervision will vary depending on the role of the clinician and the nature of the service where the work is taking place. However, the principles and techniques of psychoanalysis that are learnt during training stand the supervisor and supervisee in good stead for managing the competing demands and dynamics of NHS work. For the purposes of this chapter, I have focused on the role of service supervision in three areas: crisis work, non-specialist generic work, managing change and stress.

Supervision of crisis work

Issues of safety come up frequently in CAMHS work. Over recent years, child psychotherapists have been required to offer risk and crisis assessments. Differing sorts of risk affect young people: the risk to self (from self or others), the risk to others and the risks posed to a young person's mental health. The responsibility of clinicians in relation to these safeguarding concerns has become more defined and central to the work. CAMHS clinicians gain a lot of information and insight through their contact with a young person. They are in a position to observe their vulnerability and link with other members of a network (e.g., school, social care and family). The risks are not necessarily obvious at the outset, i.e., information suggestive of risk may only be revealed after a considerable period of getting to know the young person.

CAMHS services usually also have specialist teams that work with risk in a particular context, such as young people on the 'edge of care', where family circumstances are potentially putting the young person at risk, or those at risk of suicide, where young people's care is usually managed by specialist adolescent teams. These teams will focus not just on the mental health of the child but also on contextual factors that may contribute to risk. This approach is also essential in thinking about treatment. The treatment of young people will involve their family and network, helping to develop their understanding and change how they perceive and interact with the young person. The family and network will also be required in a more basic way to protect, support and provide safety for their child.

A particularly challenging task for clinicians is to do mental health assessments after young people present to accident and emergency (A&E) departments. CAMHS teams tend to have duty rotas of clinicians to assess young people attending hospital where a preliminary assessment has indicated mental health concerns. In the past, these assessments were not required of child psychotherapists, but this change in role has been brought about to cover the ever-increasing rate of young people attending A&E, usually having threatened or enacted self-harm or suicidal actions.

Conducting these assessments causes tension, as it is often seen as beyond the 'core role'. It is stressful and difficult work, particularly for newly qualified child psychotherapists, who have been trained in the importance of consistency and regularity. Time and space are central to containment, neither of which are available in the situation of young people attending A&E. They need assessing at short notice and at irregular times. The space in which assessments take place is usually provided ad hoc and is often not fully private. The people required for the assessment may need to be drawn in at short notice and with little time to plan.

Suicidal and self-harming young people stir up huge anxieties in everyone connected to them. Usually, they have been sent to A&E in crisis, the speed of referral for a mental health assessment also conveying the sense of the young person requiring an intensive and immediate intervention. A&E departments struggle with young people who are perhaps not seen as properly (physically) ill, coming with self-inflicted injuries or obscure thoughts of self-harm or suicide. There may be a resistance to placing a young person on a paediatric ward if they are seen to be taking the bed of someone with a more obvious (physical) affliction. They may be seen as inflicting their misfortune on themselves and so deserving of less sympathy.

If the young person has made it to a hospital ward, there can be pressure to discharge quickly. CAMHS teams are expected to keep young people out of hospital and manage them in the community. The young people themselves, and their accompanying parents, may be keen to get home, having waited for several hours to be seen and assessed. Or they may have unrealistic expectations of in-patient admission to address all their difficulties. The assessment often comes at the end of a long day – and clinicians are not paid overtime. Once a young person is seen, there will still be writing up to do.

Often the young person may resist the assessment; the desire to be heard and understood is not necessarily conscious. The family, too, may be unreceptive – displacing their anger towards their child on to the clinician, particularly if their A&E attendance seems to be at least partly the result of previously requested support from services having been refused or delayed.

Offering a sensitive and effective clinical intervention in A&E is demanding and cannot be done in isolation. It requires supervision. This is partly to help withstand the pressures and projections coming from referrers, parents and hospital services, but also to develop confidence in making robust and reliable decisions about whether it is safe to discharge, as well as to come up with sound clinical plans for a young person. The supervisor is an essential sounding board in this process. Sharing responsibility for critical safeguarding decisions allows the assessing clinician to have the confidence to explore what has gone on, to create the space and freedom to understand the young person in the context of the developmental process.

Although unwelcome and a source of dissatisfaction for many, this role is one for which child psychotherapists are well suited. A significant amount of the task is procedural, such as asking concrete questions to establish risk: the intention of the act (e.g., cutting or overdose of tablets), the intent to end life, ongoing suicidality, understanding the trigger, establishing a plan and support to ensure safety for the next 24/48/72 hours until a review can take place. However, these questions may evoke nuanced answers: a 'no' that feels like a 'yes', a sense of unease in the clinician or a feeling of disconnect or disinterest. Child psychotherapists are experienced in monitoring their counter-transference, being sensitive to feelings evoked as well as getting direct information from questions. Here again, the role of supervisor is essential in helping to explore these nuances, to give a second opinion on aspects that may have critical importance in assessing safety for discharge. By exploring unconscious as well as conscious motives and by understanding conflicts facing the young person at a particular moment in their development, child psychotherapists are well placed to offer thorough assessments that make sense of actions that seem irrational and bizarre, particularly when assessing suicidal acts. Providing a narrative that gives an explanatory framework enables an accurate assessment of risk and helps in forming a plan for successful treatment.

Clinical example 1

I feel annoyed to get the call that a young person in A&E needs to be seen, and sheepishly tell Peter (a newly qualified child psychotherapist) that he needs to go to hospital to do the assessment. It is late on a Thursday afternoon. Peter's shift was due to end at 4pm and he has plenty of other tasks to get on with. I am aware that this will be frustrating for him. The assessment will make it hard to get away on time and write it up without the work spilling over into another day when time is not allocated to complete the task.

Peter will no doubt also have to arrange a follow-up review for the young person and parent, assuming discharge from A&E is agreed. We review the case together. Alexia is a 15-year-old girl and this is her first contact with mental health services. She took 12 paracetamol tablets following an incident of cyber-bullying, in which her best friend shared information with a wide group of their social circle about a sexual encounter between Alexia and an older boy. Alexia's friend did this after they had fallen out. Peter and I think about the context of Alexia's family background – mum, stepdad and younger half-siblings – and wonder how it might be a factor in the overdose. Considering the events and the context helps us feel hopeful that the assessment will not be too complex (assuming the family environment is sufficiently safe and supportive) to be able to discharge Alexia home with a good safety plan and a review appointment date. We are also reassured that there will be an opportunity to follow up the following day (Friday), if needed. Thinking together has taken away some of the fear of the unpredictability and threat evoked by a suicidal act. It reminds us that, despite all its challenges, this is interesting work and central to our role.

Peter heads off to A&E and agrees to call me to think through any plans before decisions are made about discharge. I encourage him to call back soon because I believe collaborative thinking is essential and helps avoid getting caught up in the complex dynamics when there is risk and worry about a young person.

Peter calls me after about an hour, telling me that the overdose has stirred a tearful mum to actively engage with the difficulties her daughter is facing. Mum is outraged by the bullying and determined to protect Alexia from the attacks. She plans to get on to school to sort things out. Although Alexia had in the past complained about friendship issues, mum was unaware of the extent of the upset caused to her daughter. Mum was now going to be active in ensuring the safety of Alexia. At this point, Alexia was no longer suicidal, and discharging her home with a safety plan seemed straightforward. Her mother agreed to keep an eye on her, to oversee removing access to tablets and protecting her from other obvious dangers. Mum would keep Alexia off school for the time being and would contact school staff to address the bullying.

This might have been sufficient to address the immediate risk, however it was important to explore the wider context. Alexia's dad had left when she was five years old, following a violent relationship with mum. Alexia had intermittent contact with him until she was 12, at which point the relationship with his new family (wife and two daughters) had made things complicated. Contact became increasingly irregular until it stopped completely, causing mum indignation on Alexia's behalf.

After five years of living alone with Alexia, mum married again and had two children with Alexia's new stepdad. There was increasing conflict at home between Alexia and her stepdad. Mum described Alexia's behaviour as challenging and her own relationship with her as volatile. Although on the surface the trigger for the overdose seemed to be the bullying, it also transpired that mum and Alexia had had an argument that same day. Mum had gone out with the two half-sisters and not responded to a text message sent by Alexia.

The decision was made to discharge Alexia, but in the debrief we thought about the family dynamics and Alexia's developmental stage, caught between a wish for independence and a need for dependency. The context suggested unresolved Oedipal issues, without mum, dad or stepdad being fully available to help work these through. Alexia's siblings, like her peers, were a source of rivalry and conflict. This debrief provided clues that furthered our understanding of the suicidal act. We could then think about how best to help Alexia and her family keep her safe in the short term but also develop meaningful insight to her difficulties to support her longer term. These considerations were picked up in the follow-up review meeting and helped ensure that Alexia and her family were offered a comprehensive formulation and longer-term treatment plan, as well as an immediate safety plan.

Generic CAMHS work

A proportion of a child psychotherapist's work as a CAMHS clinician will be 'generic'. Generic work is similar across all disciplines within a multidisciplinary service. Broadly speaking, it involves initial assessments of young people coming into the service, often short-term interventions and ongoing support through 'care coordination'. In addition, there may be tasks such as risk assessments (as described above) or responding to incoming calls. Other roles may include contributing to the operational functioning of the team and carrying out administration and other tasks that relate to the quality standards of the service, all of which take up significant amounts of time.

Qualified child psychotherapists will also take on more responsibility in relation to the clinical work they are doing. Trainees have limited clinical responsibility, which is held with the service supervisor. Choices about which young people to offer child psychotherapy to, the duration of treatment or allocation of parent work will all be decided by the trainee's supervisor. If something goes wrong, it is the supervisor who has to take responsibility. The trainee's clinical notes will be validated by the supervisor, who should be aware of developments in the cases and whether there should be changes to the care plan. This enables the trainee to concentrate on their technique and the experience with the young person in therapy and gives them the freedom to build up their experience and confidence. It is quite a jump from this to the role of qualified clinician. The degree of clinical oversight and support offered by the clinical supervisor or other structures within the multi-disciplinary team will vary, but the responsibility for the clinical work will rest ultimately with the clinician themselves.

Clinical example 2

Ten-year-old Zac comes as a priority assessment, allocated to Lizzie a child psychotherapist qualified for a year. Zac has been prioritised because both parents have made frequent calls to the service with escalating worries about his behaviour. Given the long waits for assessment once a referral has been accepted, parents or members of the network may call for advice or to inform the service if there are increased risks. In Zac's case, both social care and his parents had been calling with increasing anger and agitation. The case had previously been risk assessed following an incident in which Zac pointed a knife at his mother and declared that he was going to kill himself. He was discharged with a safety plan and a referral made to social care. Because the risk of suicide was assessed as being low, he was placed back on the CAMHS waiting list for assessment.

In the weeks following the emergency assessment, Zac continued to make threats to himself and others. He threatened to climb out of a third-floor window and was aggressive to his mum, who felt she had to back down to his frequent demands. School attendance was reduced, although when he did attend, he managed well. However mum, social care and school became increasingly worried, believing that Zac had a serious mental illness. They felt that CAMHS were negligent in not considering him a high priority. Given the high level of support the case needed through telephone consultation, it was agreed that it would make sense for it to be prioritised.

A new case would normally be assessed by a single clinician and brought back for multidisciplinary discussion before a decision was made about referring for further specialist psychological therapy. The assessing clinician would be expected to 'hold' the case in the interim and to carry out ongoing work – referred to as care coordination.

In thinking about the case with Lizzie in supervision, pre-assessment, it felt important to understand the high level of anxiety that it generated, despite the fact the crisis service assessment had deemed Zac not to be risky. Social care were asking for a commitment to an offer of child psychotherapy. The pressure exerted on the clinician by the network in these circumstances can feel intense. Lizzie could foresee the challenge of managing the network and holding the line that, at least in the short term, child psychotherapy was unlikely to be suitable for Zac.

There is ongoing discussion about making use of limited clinical resources and whether it is appropriate for child psychotherapists to be offering initial assessments and care coordination rather than more specialist treatment. However, as with risk assessments, it seems important to demonstrate the unique clinical contribution that child psychotherapy can make to this sort of work, to draw attention to the skills of child psychotherapists who can be flexible in what they can offer, as well as having a particular clinical specialism.

In supervision, I remind Lizzie that, despite the challenges, there is something unique she can offer in thinking about what might be going on for Zac. However, given the circumstances of this case, it feels essential that Lizzie is joined by a second clinician to work with the network and help create the necessary space for this thinking.

We go back to the team, and it is agreed that Lizzie will be joined by a clinical nurse specialist and that the first session will be a network meeting to clarify what the assessment and initial care coordination work might look like. It is not always easy to argue for extra resources in the form of supporting clinicians when joint working is not the norm. However, in this case it is necessary to consider Zac's likely ongoing clinical needs and to avoid reaching a point where clinicians feel overwhelmed.

The presence of two clinicians in the initial network meeting was helpful in withstanding the frustration of those involved. The clinicians were struck by the force of the anger expressed but were able to articulate an initial plan for assessment as well as commit to offering further case management sessions without spelling out a longer-term plan. They were also able to communicate the aspects of support that CAMHS would *not* be able to offer, i.e., what would need to be thought about and taken up by school and social care based on the assessment and formulation.

In the assessment, the clinicians heard about Zac growing up as an only child and now living with mum, a woman in her late 40s. Dad was a significantly younger man, largely unfulfilled, living separately from mum. He had recently been drafted in to try and help her manage when Zac became aggressive. Zac struggled with separation from mum and, although he was not seen as presenting with problem behaviours at school, he continually verbalised how much he hated school and was aggressive and uncooperative in the mornings when he was due to go in. School reported that he was behind academically, and on the periphery socially. According to his mother, Zac took his anger out on her when he got home due to the stress he experienced at school. Mum felt that school had not picked up his difficulties and were not sufficiently responsive to him. She believed he was autistic and was annoyed about school's reluctance to refer him for an assessment.

Mum had allowed limited involvement from dad in Zac's upbringing, as she perceived him to be a bad influence due to his mental health difficulties and lack of engagement with Zac. Mum was exclusively the person who was on the receiving end of Zac's aggression but also the person that Zac would demand.

Lizzie described her assessment with mum and Zac, in which he would refuse to engage directly or allow separation from his mother. In response to Lizzie's comments, Zac would talk to his mother in whispers which she would relay back to Lizzie. Lizzie heard how Zac wanted to have friendships but would struggle with making consistent friends. In the last 18 months they had moved house to be near maternal grandmother, which had involved a change of school and greatly exacerbated the difficulties.

Zac presented as much younger than his ten years. Lizzie was also struck by Zac losing interest in her. He would sit on his mother's lap, playing with her long hair in a way that appeared intrusive and to Lizzie felt uncomfortable, but mum did not bat an eyelid.

Before going into further details or coming up with a detailed formulation, it is important for the CAMHS child psychotherapist involved in such assessments to consider what the task is and to think with their supervisor how best they can be supported in achieving this. At this point we do not have enough information to suggest a treatment plan. We do not know fully what other agencies are able to address or what Zac or his mum might be able to engage with. The clinician, therefore, would not have the permission (or resources) to offer a substantial piece of work, even if we think it is indicated. It is, though, possible to make use of the skills of the child psychotherapist to come to a provisional formulation that looks at the developmental and social history of the young person as well as of the clinician's experience of the child both in an individual encounter and in relation to mother.

The history suggested a failure to move towards independence from his mother at necessary points in Zac's development. There was a lack of a parental couple that might have enabled separation and moving into a post-Oedipal world in which the ordinary developments of childhood could take place. Perhaps Zac was never required to relinquish his mother and identify with his father. His behaviour in relation to his mother in the therapy room left the clinician feeling uncomfortable, and suggested something inappropriate in their relationship. Zac seemed to feel he possessed his mother sexually. We now had a basic formulation that might make sense of Zac's struggle with his peer group, his possessiveness and aggression towards mother and his struggle to accept the position of being a child who has an awareness of being dependent and not knowing things – a prerequisite to being able to learn.

We could, therefore, think of a preliminary treatment plan: fleshing out this initial formulation through further observation of Zak, and, with the support of the co-worker, supporting the family and network by offering an understanding of Zac's presentation as well as thinking about their role in helping him. Lizzie's initial sense was that his avoidance of relating to her was due to his wish to stay joined to mother, rather than being an autistic presentation. However, spending more time Zac would illuminate this further. Future contact could clarify whether there would be sufficient engagement or interest in change to indicate a more specialist intervention, such as individual psychotherapy or parent-child psychotherapy.

Clearly the degree of experience of the clinician will indicate how much support and input they need from supervision to help define these pieces of generic work. Although as experience develops less supervision is needed, it is important for all clinicians, however experienced, to have a space to discuss these cases, which can be both complex and challenging. It is the role of the supervisor to support the clinician to ensure that this work is done in a managed context, so they are not overwhelmed by the volume and complexity of the cases.

Managing change and stress

CAMHS services have undergone huge change in recent years, with the role of clinician becoming more complex and stressful. Increasing oversight and scrutiny, along with demands to demonstrate efficacy, generate extra tasks which reduce the time available for direct clinical work. For example, as well as documenting concerns about risk that may be picked up in the course of their work, clinicians are required to contribute to ongoing safeguarding concerns through the framework of Child Protection Planning and Child in Need meetings. They are also expected to contribute to processes in schools, through Educational Health Care Planning, advocating for other educational and emotional support and contributing to discussions about suitable school placements. Meanwhile, continuing financial constraints have led to a pressure to create efficiency savings through rationalisation and retendering. One consequence of this has been services moving into more 'efficient' premises, often with reductions in clinical space (such as dedicated rooms for child psychotherapy), or the use of open plan 'hot-desking' office environments.

The legacy of Covid

These ongoing and incremental changes were evident before the impact of the Covid pandemic, which has caused monumental shifts in clinical and work-based practice, including uses of technology, the offer of remote sessions, changes in clinical technique, meeting arrangements and the social and interactive experience of work, as well as the legacy of the direct impact of Covid on families and clinicians. Such changes present significant challenges and generate huge anxiety, therefore requiring considerable space in supervision. One example was the expectation during the early stages of the pandemic that all clinicians would be on a rota to offer face-to-face appointments to young people in crisis. Worries about contracting Covid were compounded by lack of clarity about protective measures and levels of risk for clinicians from different demographics. Some were required to make risky journeys to get to work, whereas others who lived more locally were able to attend with less perceived risk. Some clinicians were frustrated by the lack of opportunity to offer clinical work (particularly trainees keen to complete casework, much of which was not possible to do remotely), whereas others were reluctant to attend clinic for fear of putting themselves and their families at risk.

The role of the supervisor inevitably entails containing the clinician in these circumstances, creating space for reflection both in individual supervisions and within the team process. Uncertainty and change generate anger, and those in senior roles are frequently on the receiving end of frustration and dissatisfaction. The supervisor needs to hold on to the reasoning for the 'corporate position' but also recognise the experience of loss and fear that these changes involve. This requires some acceptance of responsibility (on behalf of the organisation) for the change, as a senior clinician has more influence to affect how the service can respond to it. It is difficult to achieve a balance, given the temptation to join with the complaints, which are often justified, whilst trying to help process an experience of loss, as well as challenging operational changes that are ill-advised or unsafe. Senior clinicians in a supervisory role who link to both clinical work and management process are well placed to do this but need good supervision of their own if they are to be effective.

Complaints and serious incidents

Another source of pressure for clinicians comes from increasing numbers of complaints and serious incidents. Serious incidents usually involve the death of a child, or a near miss which requires investigation. Complaints by parents about specific clinicians or services in general also lead to investigations. Evidence suggests that the frequency of these incidents and complaints is growing, to the point where most clinicians will be subjected to them at some point. I have supervised many clinicians who have been on the receiving end of such investigations. Whilst the impact will vary depending on the seriousness of the incident, it is inevitably extremely stressful for clinicians to be faced with the feelings caused by the event itself and by the investigation.

Usually the investigations are managed sensitively, but there is, nonetheless, an onus on the service to demonstrate that something has been learned from the incident, with the implication that mistakes were made. Clinical notes are explored, which may highlight gaps or areas for improvement. Perceived imperfections may well be brought up in reviews, compounding feelings of failure and guilt about the incident and creating intense anxiety.

Supervision is essential in these circumstances, providing ongoing space for the incident to be reviewed and thought about. The responsibility held by the supervisor is also important in helping to mitigate the impact on the clinician. The recognition of our limits as clinicians is central to this, i.e., challenging omnipotence is crucial. Working with children necessarily involves responsibility and, therefore, a burden of feelings if things go wrong. Part of the supervisor's role can be to support the clinician in challenging the outcome or tone of a report. However, it is also important to take time to explore the details of the case, away from an official explanation, to understand what might have happened. This is where going back to a psychoanalytic formulation and considering not only the circumstances of the incident but also the process and system around the investigation can provide the space to make sense of the clinician's experience. This can facilitate their learning from the incident and also help them process the trauma.

Conclusion

My aim in this chapter has been to convey a sense of the complexity of working in CAMHS the range of clinical and organisational skills required and the role of the service supervisor in supporting the child psychotherapist through this. Such complexity is hard for one person to manage without reference to a clinical supervisor who can assist in thinking through the different roles and responsibilities. Child psychotherapists train to do child psychotherapy out of an interest in the theory and technique and a belief in the power of the treatment. It is essential for the flourishing of the profession that space is made in CAMHS for this clinical specialism. It is also essential to advocate for children and young people with complex emotional needs to access psychotherapy; such children need time and space for the slow unfurling of internal conflicts within the unfolding transference relationship.

However, to maintain the demand for child psychotherapists within CAMHS, it is also essential that clinicians adapt to the other roles that are now required. In my experience, child psychotherapists are sought-after clinicians, bringing their specialist skills and insights to generic tasks and case formulations. Similarly, their understanding of group process helps facilitate team functioning and the work with complex networks and families which is a staple of clinical work.

Supervision plays a vital role in helping the clinician preserve their specialism while also finding meaning and enjoyment in generic work. Given the demands on all clinicians in the ever-changing world of child and adolescent mental health in the NHS, supervision is also essential in providing space to recognise the limits of the clinical role and to push back when the expectations are unrealistic, or the impact of the changes are unmanageable. Maintaining this balance will help ensure that child psychotherapists continue to make a vital contribution to the mental health of young people treated in the public sector.

Chapter 6

How can I put this?

Writing as supervision

Julie Kitchener

For clinicians so attuned to the psychic value of play and playfulness, child psychotherapists spend a lot of time hunched at their desks 'writing up' – file notes,
reports, letters, presentations ... those copious 'process' notes we labour over after
sessions, and which form the basis of most case supervisions both pre- and post-
qualification. Writing about what we do is an inescapable part of what we do, perhaps more so since the medium has morphed from paper to screen. How has this
come about? What, or who, is all this writing for?

Freud, of course, took the written word extremely seriously. 'If we could at
least discover in ourselves or in people like ourselves an activity which was
in some way akin to writing', he muses in his 1908 essay 'Creative writers
and day-dreaming' (S Freud [1907]1908: 143). References to literature, from
Shakespeare to Terry Pratchett, have permeated the pages of psychoanalysis
ever since. 'Writing', argues the American psychoanalyst Thomas Ogden, 'is a
unique form of thinking' (Ogden 2012: 7). Freud himself, Ann Horne reminds
us, wrote 'simply, clearly and extremely well' ([2011]2019: 156). Other 'masters
of language' have followed (Hayman 2013: 63), and not necessarily confined to
any one theoretical tradition – though it could be argued, as Adam Phillips suggests, that what used to be called the Middle Group is distinguished from the
other psychoanalytic trainings by its 'distinctive writers' rather than a shared
ideology: 'an unofficial version of psychoanalysis, in the best sense' (Phillips
2021: 96). Indeed, Winnicott, notoriously too independent to consider himself
an Independent, left a literary legacy that Ogden has likened to 'prose poems'
(Ogden 2012: 76).

Not all psychoanalytic writing is so readable. Nor is there a straightforward
equation between 'good' writing (whatever we think that is) and clinical skill or
analytic insight. And, anyway, few child psychotherapists enter the profession with
a view to becoming a Writer, despite the growing interest in the ethics and practice of clinical and research publishing in recent years. Why, then, do our trainings and supervisions keep us so tied to our keyboards? Was Freud right: can the
activity of writing – and those skilled in its craft – teach us something about being
a psychotherapist?

DOI: 10.4324/9781003297604-8

Naming and framing

'Jordan' leans over the sink where all his animals float. 'I know, let's play ...' He attempts to explain but can't seem to get anything going. He says a word, rejects it, attempts another but rejects that too. All the while, he flings himself on to the chair, leaps up, hurries to the sink, then back again. No, he tells me, he can't start, he wants me to. I say, ok, but I'm going to start by describing what I can see and add what I think might be going on.

'Ok.' Jordan scurries over to stand by me, clutching the rim of the sink.

'Once upon a time ...' I begin. Jordan grins. 'There was a little lamb afloat on a big pool –'

'Sea,' Jordan hisses from behind his hand.'Oh, ok. Sorry. I mean on a huge sea ... An ocean, in fact.'

Jordan's grin broadens. Then he says excitedly, 'I'll do the actions and you have to say what you see.' He splashes around the lamb's boat.

And so the story continues ...

A supervisor's eye might catch in this vignette the therapist's shift from 'subjective object' (Winnicott 1971a: 4) to 'auxiliary ego' (A Freud 1965: 42–43) or wonder about the chaos of seven-year-old Jordan's inner world, the anxiety expressed in his bodily propulsion. But my interest for the moment is the way the sequence parallels the process of writing. From a structural point of view, we see Jordan's struggle to give form to his thoughts, to make sense of an emotional and physical experience, the flood of his 'affect storms' (McDougall 1984: 400). In response, the therapist (me, let's say) offers the scaffolding of the conventional story form. Likewise, process notes can help shape even the most chaotic clinical material. Whether through pen, keyboard or voice-recognition, once our notes start appearing 'out there', in black and white, on paper/on screen, we have a chance to step back and take a view of a session, to think beginning, middle and end, to feel less overwhelmed. Writing becomes a way of ordering experience, enabling us to 'ride the emotional spectrum', as poet and 'artist of languages' Nicki Jackowska puts it. 'But filtered, sifted, whittled and directed' (1997: 39).

Maria Rhode, a wise and generous supervisor in her own right, has argued the value of process notes as 'an enactment of a three-party constellation', an important first supervision, particularly in work with highly disturbed patients (Rhode 1998: 231–242). She describes how writing up her notes on an intensely challenging session with a young autistic boy allowed her to make sense of a sequence that had been incomprehensible to her in the room, the power of her patient's projections having left her mind 'literally in pieces'. Even if the 'third party is no more than a piece of paper', Rhode says, it offers the therapist an Oedipal perspective, a reinstatement of 'the analyst's internal reflective relationship with his or her own analytic function' (Rhode 1998: 241). Freud undoubtedly understood this third-party aspect of writing (though maybe not its supervisory potential). As Ogden shows in his essay on 'Mourning and melancholia', when we read Freud, 'we can see a great deal of thinking is occurring in the very act of writing a few words' (Ogden 2012: 7). For Rhode, the act of writing created a space for thought which, in turn, enabled her to re-establish contact with her patient and therapeutic work to progress.

Say what you see

'Something about a situation will bother me', the novelist and essayist Joan Didion once told *The Paris Review*, 'so I will write a piece to find out what it is that bothers me.'[1] Rhode was bothered, and in bothering to write up her patient's session she was surprised by a moment of clinical insight. This insight was prompted, you could say, by her discovering as she wrote 'what was in fact lying around waiting to be found' (Winnicott [1963]1965: 181). From this Winnicottian perspective, taking the trouble to write up can facilitate the creative processes of therapy, offering opportunities for surprise. Gail Phillips, in conversation with Mani Vastardis about their supervisions together, notes how from this 'triangulated position' a therapist often 'stumbles across things, overlooked in the session, but which seem to leap off the page' (Vastardis and Phillips 2012: 119).

According to Louis MacNeice, 'the poet's first business is *mentioning* things'.[2] So too, perhaps, for the child psychotherapist. From our first infant observation, as nascent trainees, we are encouraged to follow Jordan's injunction to 'say what you see'. As MacNeice knew – as we discover – there is more to this apparently effortless notion than meets the eye. 'You know', a trainee recounts during supervision,

> it was only when I wrote this up that I realised what I'd seen. In fact, when Charlie rattled off all that stuff about how helpful her sessions were and what a good holiday she'd had, she also pushed up her sleeves, like she was preparing for a fight. It was then I must have noticed the scars.

Like Rhode, the trainee writing her process notes discovers she has 'seen' something she had not processed at the time. It almost escaped mention.

The American author Anne Lamott maintains that writing itself hones the attention, it 'motivates you to look closely at life' (Lamott 1995: xii). Close attention is not tunnel vision, though it carries that risk. Constraints on perception and emotional availability have been highlighted in the debate around the impact of remote working on the therapeutic encounter – the limits of screen vision – but even in the room what we notice will depend on the always inevitable distractibility of our 'evenly suspended attention' (S Freud 1912: 111), so often drawn in the direction of desire and expectation. 'Somehow those scars didn't register', Charlie's therapist admits. 'I was so taken up with how positive she was being about her progress.'

Whatever dominates the foreground, attuning to unconscious processes requires a capacity for varifocal perception, shifting between close up and periphery, learning to 'say what we see' without rushing to file it under 'understood' or 'just what I was looking for'. There are parallels here with the observational skills cultivated by nature writers. Kathleen Jamie, whose poetry and prose are so evocative of the landscapes of Scotland, describes the challenge of allowing herself 'to notice, but not to analyse ... to hush the frantic inner voice that says, "Don't be stupid," and learn again to look, to listen' (Jamie 2005: 42).

Truth and fiction

'We make it all up, anyway, don't we?' a supervisee suggests, not entirely tongue in cheek. She has a point. Giving shape to our thoughts on paper can, paradoxic- ally, make us unreliable narrators. 'We know that the first step towards attaining intellectual mastery of our environment is to discover generalizations, rules and laws which bring order into chaos', Freud tells us in 'Analysis terminable and interminable'. 'In doing this we simplify the world of phenomena; but we cannot avoid falsifying it, especially if we are dealing with processes of development and change' (S Freud 1937: 228). However tenuously, Jordan and I were attempting to find meaning in his mayhem; a process that necessarily requires focus and filter. This may or may not have been appropriate clinically, but in my attempts to record and order the experience afterwards – to save myself as well as little lamb from drowning – I created a brief and rather tidy narrative.

To be fair, the vignette from Jordan's session was an extract, not the full write- up. An alternative version could have included, for argument's sake, a giraffe in a noose, a de-antlered stag, a tap wrenched on, a plug plunged into place, water gushing and spattering, Jordan humming and 'psss-ing' in imitation (the devil is in the detail), my irritation; it could have continued with a voyage of capsizings, near drownings, thwarted attempts at rescue, a drenched carpet ... Would all this have escaped the process of selection? Probably not. The analyst who writes down a session, note the Swedish psychoanalysts Johan Norman and Björn Salomonsson, 'inevitably makes choices. Different aspects are felt to be avoided, evocative, attractive, etc, depending on the analyst's thinking, training, experience and per- sonality' (Norman and Salomonsson 2005: 1295).

'You have to keep getting out of your own way so that whatever it is that wants to be written can use you to write it', counsels Lamott (1995: 8). Which takes us back to free-associative basics. Freud's idea of an activity 'in some ways akin' to that of creative writers, was in part influenced by an essay by Karl Ludwig Börne (1786–1837), 'The art of becoming an original writer in three days'. Freud quotes Börne's recommendation to write down 'without any falsification or hypocrisy, everything that comes into your head' (S Freud 1920: 265). According to Freud's 'Fundamental Technical Rule', as every analysand and analyst knows, this includes those details that might feel 'disagreeable', 'nonsensical', 'unimportant' or 'irrele- vant to what is being looked for' (S Freud [1922]1923: 238).

Hard enough to achieve on the couch; even more of a challenge in our write-ups. Which is why we learn to cultivate – or at least tolerate – the supervisor (internal or external) who nags for that little bit more from our notes: 'What led up to that?' 'Where were you sitting?' 'What colour crayon did she choose?' There is another form of 'making it up': the attempt to bring experience to life through the telling. The story of Jordan's therapy is evoked through its details: the regression in his splashing, the impotence of the de-antlered stag, the entanglement with his object, the annihilatory near drownings ...

It is 'the real detail', argues the poet and teacher Peter Sansom, describing a poem by Simon Armitage, 'which makes it "true" ... unsentimental and written plainly, simply, just as it was seen' (Sansom 1994: 9). We can't all be poets, even if our patients offer up some of our best lines, but we can expand our mentioning skills.

A plea for a measure of incoherence

If mentioning is an art, still we try to discover its science. All that fretting during our observations and training ... When is the best time to do your write-up? What if there's no space between sessions to get anything down? (There never is.) How do you remember exactly what the child said, what you said, the specific order in which things happened? We want to capture and preserve 'like a bowlful of blue water – mustn't spill a drop' (Jamie 2005: 41), to re-create whole sessions that encapsulate our understanding of this child and their therapy.

'[U]nfortunately, I cannot give the sequence which nevertheless I am quite sure is significant', shrugs Winnicott ([1949]1958: 249). Ever alert to restrictive prac- tices, Winnicott understood 'the cohesion of ideas' as a 'defence organisation', just as 'free association that reveals a coherent theme is already affected by anx- iety' (Winnicott 1971b: 65). Indeed, the story that so often impinges on our ability to 'say what we see' is one of anxious allegiance, a misguided search for what we perceive as psychoanalytic 'truth' – or our teachers' psychoanalytic truth. 'Oh, Julie, you are being *good*', my supervisor smiles. She knows my carefully worked Kleinian script of a session suits neither me nor my four-year-old patient, at least in this instance – even if it works for her. 'Now, tell me again, what exactly hap- pened there?'

Dogma and orthodoxy make clumsy censors, particularly in the early stages of training when we are so keen to 'get it right'. Even as clinical experience teaches the therapeutic value of tact, timing and pragmatism, we invoke the tyranny of the perfect write-up, feeling like cheats when we scrabble together notes from one of yesterday's sessions because we forgot it was our turn to present in the clinical seminar today. 'It's not very well written', we say, or 'I did everything wrong, as you'll see ...', when, in fact, the hardest challenge for a supervisor can be tracing the to-and-fro of session material packed into finely polished process notes. Unlike a novelist or a poet, a psychotherapist's best write-up is likely to be their first and only draft.

A supervisee says, 'I'm not quite sure where this came', or 'I really can't remember when the ambulance got smashed', or 'At some point the baby ended up on the dolls' house roof'. He conveys the dreamlike quality of the experience, the non-linearity of unconscious communication, what may be lost or found in secondary revision. I notice too, though, that he tends always to bring this child's Monday sessions. Yes, he agrees, that has occurred to him. It is the one he knows he'll have time to write up straight afterwards. We consider timetable pressures, the challenge of the material, his fear of something being missed if he leaves too big a gap and other children start to crowd into his mind ...

Could he, I wonder, occasionally leave his writing up till later? Process notes might also benefit from slack: if not quite John Keats's 'diligent indolence' (1819), at least what the novelist Jesse Greengrass described, in an essay brilliantly subtitled the 'Intersection of muse and routine', that ' "sleight of hand" called *doing other things*' (Greengrass 2022, emphasis in original). Walking, gardening, washing-up even – anything that leaves space for the mind to roam, for session material to mull itself over, make its own links, free from scrutiny.

Maybe, the supervisee says, he'll bring Wednesday's write-up next time – 'though it won't be very good'.

The sense in a sentence

'[H]itch your unconscious mind to your writing arm,' advises Dorothea Brande in her classic *Becoming a Writer* (1934: 69). She is not advocating personal analysis, simply cultivating that working relationship between psyche and soma we tend to call 'practice'. We may be losing the tangible engagement of hand and pen (and there are good arguments for note-writing by hand, not least the absence of cut and paste and iCloud storage), but our words still reach the page through our thinking, feeling bodies.

'I wish these pages could sulk, cry, or scream', rails Björn Salomonsson (2018: 172), conveying in that brief sentence the sensory force of parent-infant work, the challenge to capture preverbal experience in words. A trainee interrupts her presentation to say: 'What I've written doesn't come close to the intensity of what was happening in the room.' She had struggled to find the right words. But her struggle was the point. Writing is hard work. Jordan hurls himself around the room, as if a train of thought might fly from his hurtling form. 'I'll do the actions,' becomes the way he shares his story with his therapist. A good sentence 'breathes and moves like a living thing', writes social and cultural historian Joe Moran. 'It is words set in motion' (Moran 2018: 26). If a child can evoke a visceral response in us (call it counter-transference), is it possible for our notes to do the same?

The child psychotherapist Hamish Canham in his exploration of Seamus Heaney's poems of childhood, considers the question of how poets put 'feeling into words'. 'The other side of this', writes Canham, 'is of putting *feelings* into words.' He argues that 'as it were', you feel the words as you write, 're-experiencing in the act of writing or reading the original sensation which led to the idea' (Canham 2003: 194, emphasis in original). As I write up Jordan's session, I am once again immersed in the plunging, gushing, spattering. I notice the shift from 'pool', to 'sea', to 'ocean'. I note, too, the 'pss' in 'sea', the hush I introduce with 'ocean' ... 'Words have halos, patinas, overhangs, echoes', says short story writer Donald

Bartheleme (1987: 21). It is their relationships that give them their momentum, their life; the links that they bring, and the way that we join them together.

The word 'sentence', Joe Moran points out, carries its own echoes, deriving from the Latin *sentire* – to feel – but also denoting a judicial verdict. When we write up our notes, we are engaged in Winnicott's 'highly specialized form of playing in the service of communication with oneself and others' (1971b: 48). To convey meaning, writing requires judgement as well as feeling. Like the analytic frame, its forms and conventions can protect and facilitate creative processes, even as (and often because) we kick against their constraints.

As Moran says,

> Rules force us to plumb our brain's depths for the word that will fit the shape it needs to fit. They let us say things that are just beyond our imaginative reach and write over our own heads before we know quite what we are saying.
>
> (Moran 2018: 27)

Whose words are they, anyway?

Rules, of course, also create barriers. 'How do you spell failure?' asks nine-year-old Stevie, reminding me that the written word can exclude as well as embrace. 'I wish I could destroy all the paper in the world', she adds, ''cos if we didn't have paper, there wouldn't be any learning.' Another day, she says, 'I like school, but there's this thing I don't like – what's it called? – Reading. Yeah. Reading. I don't like that … Or writing.'

A trainee takes a session to supervision that she recorded last night through her mobile phone. If it wasn't for voice recognition technology, she says, she's not sure she'd have made it on to the training. ('I was amazed at how easy writing is if you take away spelling and grammar. If you just say it', recalled the journalist A A Gill, in his ferocious account of his experience of dyslexia within the British social and educational system ([2010]2017: 365).

A supervising psychotherapist facilitating a regular work discussion group of mental health professionals notices that one member, a highly skilled clinician, never presents. After a while it dawns on the facilitator to suggest that full session notes might not be necessary *every* week. Immediately, the clinician asks to bring some material. The following week he introduces the group to mind maps – spider's web diagrams that ignite the discussion with new free-associative energy. Independent trainings may be less inclined to process note policing – indeed Balint groups have never required written presentations – but supervisors make assumptions borne of their background, experience and relationship to writing.

Issues of power, privilege and exclusion are written through our professions, despite recent changes designed to make them more inclusive and representative of the communities they serve. Writing itself sits at that 'the grim intersection of class, race, disability and gender' (de Waal 2019: xi). While the boundaries within the world of publishing are becoming more porous, anyone working with unconscious processes knows that the rules of exclusion can be internalised as well as manifest. Nobel Laureate Toni Morrison highlighted the black writer's need to resist 'the white gaze' – the assumed white reader of fiction (Morrison 1992). The Scottish writer, activist and rapper Darren McGarvey has described working with marginalised young people, 'trying to explain to them … you always have this idea that people like me don't write, you know, you put a pen and paper down and they just interpret it as stress'.[3]

I ask a group of trainee child psychotherapists during a clinical seminar how many of them feel anxious when they know it is their turn to present. Everyone. I wonder why they think that might be. One volunteers the familiar fear of being judged, prompting a collective nodding. Another adds: 'I worry my notes won't do justice to my patient.' Like the children we work with, our notes cannot escape the sociopolitical dynamics played out through language, on and off the page. But being open to a child's experience also means recognising that our process notes are a form of co-creation; it is our patients who inspire and inhabit the words we use. 'Each child has his own theory', writes the French analyst Catherine Mathelin, 'and it is from him that we get it' (1994: 18).

Vital clues and a musical ear

Supervisor: Listen to how your patient hears what you say.
Child: This is you saying, "Oh, Jordan's doing this; Jordan's doing that"

We write up and then we read out loud. An odd thing for an adult to do. Farhad Dalal describes, with incisive humour, an early experience of supervision:

> The first part of each supervision consisted of me reading out my notes from my notebook, and whilst I did this the supervisor wrote down what I was reading out into his notebook. About two thirds of the way though the 50-minute session, he would then tell me what had really been taking place in my therapy session. This I duly and dutifully wrote down into my notebook.
>
> (Dalal 2021: 5)

Supervision by dictation: the superego sabotage of voice and ear, reducing a lived encounter to 'the dried minestrone of speech' (Gill [2010]2017: 360). Novelists and poets know that they work with the voice 'warm from the mouth', as Gill puts it. Reading out loud returns words to the body, enables writer and listener to test their resonance. Too much focus on the visual text in supervision stifles exchange and conversation, renders us oblivious to sense and nuance, to the pace of the therapeutic work, the idiom of patient and therapist.

A trainee sits tense and upright opposite his supervisor, reading robotically through his notes on a particularly difficult session with a 12-year-old – she did this, I did that – until he reaches a passage where the girl describes her fear that she might vomit. 'So I tell her,' the trainee recounts, slipping into his more natural speaking voice, '"I think you've been throwing up plenty here – and you haven't got rid of me yet."' The girl appears to ignore him, launching into a familiar recount of past events, only there's an extra element of experiential detail, her distress tangible in the tone of her therapist's reading voice. The supervisor notices this shift with the trainee, the fluctuation of tenses as he presented, from distanced reporting to immediate exchange, the subtle change effected in his patient.

'The original experience of primitive agony', says Winnicott, 'cannot get into the past tense unless the ego can first gather it into its own present time experience' ([1963?]1974: 91). Perhaps, particularly when trauma threatens to overwhelm, the presence of the supervisor can echo the 'presence of the therapist' (Lanyado 2004). Tone and timbre – the voice as a 'sound-object', as Susan Maello has described it (1995) – are, then, integral to the creation of a facilitating supervisory environment, allowing us to re-read and reprocess. The supervisor who adopts a 'poetic stance' (Yerushalmi 2021: 116), who, as Maello suggests, listens with a 'musical ear', can enhance our capacity to give voice to our patients' experience. In the process, we sharpen our listening skills, tune into a wider variety of voices, notice our deaf spots, discover different ways of 'speaking' with our patients, find our own therapeutic voice. We might even take pleasure in this reading aloud of our notes, gesture blending with symbol, words reverberating between reader and listener.

'Whouff!!' a child psychotherapist veers backwards as she reads, arm raised, reliving the way she fielded the comment her teenaged patient had just hurled at her. 'Whouff!' her clinical group smile, catching the interpretive nature of her gesture, the unconscious communication between the two. 'Yeah,' her patient laughs. 'Take that, you stupid therapist.' He holds out a hand for her return throw. She answers with a gentle lob.

A confusion of tongues

'English is getting nounier', complains Moran (2018: 58), protesting against the increasing dominance of compacted official language and technical jargon – language that may be useful for conceptualisation in science and academia, but which becomes meaningless in real-life human interaction. 'In nouny writing, anything can be claimed and nothing can be felt', Moran argues. The Independent analyst Anne Hayman made a similar point 50 years ago, when she identified the risks and categorical confusions that can result in psychoanalytic thinking from the reification of abstract terms, the slippage between the language necessary for theoretical conceptualisation and that used in clinical description (Hayman 2013: Chapter 8).

  If psychoanalytic terminology can lend itself to concrete thinking, so too can the closed language of mental health bureaucracy – language whose distance from human experience would have been familiar to Franz Kafka. As Moran says, 'We act like verbs, not nouns' (2018: 57), and process notes are intrinsically more verb than noun. But such an approach to clinical writing does not translate easily into audit and data collection, the 'performance reporting' Briggs (2018: 174–175) suggests is the most accurate way to describe 'what is taken to be supervision' in Child and Adolescent Mental Health Services (CAMHS).

What role for detailed write-ups, when there is so little time for individual case supervision, because 'concentration is on the clinician's bureaucratic tasks, and not tasks that are about understanding the clinical relationship with the patient' (Briggs 2018)? This is not an argument against good management – of behaving ourselves as well as being ourselves (see Horne, Chapter 1). It is important that child psychotherapists and their supervisors find ways to negotiate the tension between the needs of their patients and the administrative demands of the service (see Daltrop, Chapter 5), just as issues of consent to publish and data protection have, quite rightly, heightened attention to the rights of patients and clients over what is recorded or published about them. There is no substitute for simple, clear, well-written file notes and reports.

Good management, then, is an argument for minding the language we use when writing about our patients. If our psychoanalytic training encourages us to interrogate and evolve our writing practice, we may be in a better position to help our patients' voices to be heard through the din of acronym-speak that crowds their 'mental health' files. The detailed session notes we take to individual case supervision are 'not an unequivocal chain of indisputable events' (Norman and Salomonsson 2005: 1283), nor, in themselves, a record of success or failure. Instead, writing up draws our attention to the shifts and fluctuations, the flow and counterflow, the lulls and jolts that are the process of a session, the process of a therapy – the process of a therapist's development. It is our internalisation of this creative supervisory experience, rather than the apparatus of file and record, that, in the end, makes us useful to our patients. After that, it is a question of Winnicott's 'riddance' (Reeves 1996).

'Julie, stop,' Jordan pulls the plug on little lamb's adventures and flops back on the chair.
'We're doing a game with less words now.'

Notes

1 The Art of Nonfiction. No. 1. Interview with Hilton Als, *Paris Review* Issue 176. Spring 2006
2 MacNeice, L (1938: 5) *Modern Poetry: A Personal Essay* Oxford: Oxford
3 Start the Week, BBC Radio 4 Monday 13 June 2022

References

Bartheleme, D (1987) Not knowing. In Kim Herzinger (ed.) *Not Knowing: The Essays and Interviews of Donald Barthelme* New York: Random House, 1997.
Brande, D (1934) *Becoming a Writer* London and Basingstoke: Papermac/Pan Macmillan, 1983.

Briggs, A (2018) Containment lost: the challenge to child psychotherapists posed by modern CAMHS. *Journal of Child Psychotherapy 44 (2)*: 168–180.

Canham, H (2003) 'Feeling into words': evocations of childhood in the poems of Seamus Heaney. In Hamish Canham and Carole Satyamurti (eds.) *Acquainted with the Night: Psychoanalysis and the Poetic Imagination* Abingdon: Routledge.

Dalal, F (2021) The ethics of supervision: reciprocity, emergence and prefiguration. *Group Analysis* Sage Journals doi:https://doi.org/10.1177/05333164211050756.

de Waal, K (2019) Foreword. In K de Waal (ed.) *Common People: An Anthology of Working-Class Writers* London: Unbound.

Freud, A (1965) *Normality and Pathology in Childhood: Assessments of Development* London: Hogarth Press.

Freud, S ([1907]1908) Creative writers and day-dreaming *SE IX* London: Vintage.

Freud, S (1912) Recommendations to physicians practising psycho-analysis *SE XII* London: Vintage, 2001.

Freud, S (1920) A note on the pre-history of the technique of analysis *SE XVIII* London: Vintage.

Freud, S ([1922]1923) Two encyclopaedia articles (A) Psycho-analysis *SE XVIII* London: Vintage.

Freud, S (1937) Analysis terminable and interminable *SE XXIII* London: Vintage.

Gill, A A ([2010] 2017) Dyslexia. In *The Best of A A Gill* London: Weidenfeld & Nicholson.

Greengrass, J (2022) Learning, practice and repetition: why the act of writing is work. Literary Hub January 5 https://lithub.com/learning-practice-and-repetition-why-the-act-of-writing-is-work.

Hayman, A (2013) *What Do Our Terms Mean? Explorations Using Psychoanalytic Theories and Concepts* London: Karnac.

Horne, A ([2011]2019) Towards a voice of one's own. In *On Children Who Privilege the Body: Reflections of an Independent Psychotherapist* Abingdon: Routledge.

Jackowska, N (1997) *Write for Life: How to Inspire Your Creative Writing* Shaftesbury: Element Books.

Jamie, K (2005) *Findings* London: Sort Of Books.

Keats, J (1819) 19 March journal letter to George and Georgiana Keats. In Hyder E Rollins (ed.) *The Letters of John Keats 1814–1821*, Volume *II* Cambridge University Press

Lamott, A (1995) *Bird by Bird: Some Instructions on Writing and Life* New York: Anchor Books.

Lanyado, M (2004) *The Presence of the Therapist: Treating Childhood Trauma* Hove: Brunner-Routledge.

McDougall, J (1984) The 'dis-affected' patient': reflections on affect pathology. *Psychoanalytic Quarterly 53*: 386–409.

Maello, S (1995) The sound-object: a hypothesis about prenatal auditory experience and memory. *Journal of Child Psychotherapy 21 (1)*: 23–41.

Mathelin, C (1994) *The Broken Piano, Lacanian Psychotherapy with Children* New York: The Other Press.

Moran, J (2018) *First You Write a Sentence: The Elements of Reading, Writing … and Life* Penguin Random House.

Morrison, T (1992) *Playing in the Dark: Whiteness and the Literary Imagination* New York: Vintage Books.

Norman, J and Salomonsson, B (2005) 'Weaving thoughts': a method for presenting and commenting on psychoanalytic case material in a peer group. *International Journal of Psychoanalysis 86*: 1281–1298.

Ogden, T H (2012) *Creative Readings: Essays on Seminal Analytic Works* Hove: Routledge.

Phillips, A (2021) *The Cure for Psychoanalysis* London: Confer Books.

Reeves, C (1996) Transition and transience: Winnicott on leaving and dying. *Journal of Child Psychotherapy 22 (3)*: 444–455.

Rhode, M (1998) Some aspects of dependence on the therapist's mental functioning. *Journal of Melanie Klein and Object Relations 16 (2)*: 233–243.

Salomonsson, B (2018) *Psychodynamic Interventions in Pregnancy and Infancy: Clinical and Theoretical Perspectives* Abingdon and New York: Routledge.

Sansom, P (1994) *Writing Poems* Newcastle Upon Tyne: Bloodaxe Books.

Vastardis, M and Phillips, G (2012) On psychoanalytic supervision: avoiding omniscience, encouraging play. In A Horne and M Lanyado (eds.) *Winnicott's Children* Hove: Routledge.

Winnicott, D W ([1949]1958) Mind and its relation to the psyche-soma. In *Through Paediatrics to Psychoanalysis: Collected Papers* London: Hogarth.

Winnicott, D W ([1963]1965) Communicating and not communicating leading to a study of certain opposites. In *The Maturational Processes and the Facilitating Environment* London: Karnac Books.

Winnicott, D W ([1963?]1974) Fear of breakdown. In C Winnicott, R Shepherd, M Davis (eds.) *Psycho-Analytic Explorations* Cambridge, MA: Harvard University Press.

Winnicott, D W (1971a) Introduction. In *Therapeutic Consultations in Child Psychiatry* New York: Basic Books.

Winnicott, D W (1971b) Playing: the search for self. In *Playing and Reality* Harmondsworth: Penguin.

Yerushalmi, H (2021) Authentic voices in supervision. *British Journal of Psychotherapy 37 (1)*: 116–129.

Part 2

Broadening horizons

Chapter 7

Supervision in extraordinary times

Teresa Bailey

A principal expectation of supervision is that we help the child psychotherapist adapt to changing demands from the environment to best meet the needs of the child. One of the starkest and most challenging recent events was the pandemic. This chapter was written during Covid and illustrates the pressures that both the supervisor and the child psychotherapist faced.

The broader context

Since the worldwide outbreak of the Covid pandemic the world has had to adapt to new ways of living and working. Public health, business, education, the National Health Service (NHS), political and societal shifts have determined new contexts in which work takes place. These have had profound effects on how we provide clinical work and also how we engage in supervision, effects that may or may not prove permanent in some respects.

When I refer to supervision, I am thinking of clinical supervision provided by senior child psychotherapists in the NHS and in private practice, to both trainee and qualified child psychotherapists and clinical managers in senior positions in NHS trusts where their work spans leadership and management roles. However, I think much of what I have written can apply to those professionals outside the health service to whom we offer consultation: in education, health, social care, the youth criminal justice system, for example. It can also apply to service managers and administrative staff, both groups to which senior child psychotherapists may find themselves providing consultation.

At the time of writing, Covid is still causing deaths and serious illness, so we continue to exist in extraordinary times, with a new Covid variant spreading quickly around the world, borders closing once more, face coverings becoming mandatory again in shops and on public transport. Many in the UK have now been vaccinated, including teenagers and some children, but we have also learned of the deaths of children from Covid when, for the last year or so, the many thousands of deaths were associated with older, vulnerable adults.

The pandemic rocked many organisations, including the NHS, forcing ongoing strategies, priorities and plans off the agenda as managers and clinicians have tried

DOI: 10.4324/9781003297604-10

to deal with rapidly changing rules. Remote working has become the norm. Online meetings – clinical and management – therapy and supervision over Zoom have become part of everyday practice. Staff well-being has needed to assume much greater attention than it may have done prior to the pandemic in order to prevent splits developing in teams and services as some staff reportedly refused the vaccine and mask wearing and even challenged whether Covid is real.

In addition to workplace concerns, isolation, illness and working from home, political and societal shifts have also had a huge impact, since the beginning of 2020. The Metropolitan Police have been accused of institutional misogyny, having already been declared institutionally racist. The undermining of our sense of safety, and our faith in institutions, has aggravated the frightening effects of Covid. Shock waves still reverberate across society as we have been confronted with the horror of the filmed murder of George Floyd. Movements such as 'Me Too', 'Black Lives Matter', Trans rights campaigns, the Climate Emergency, Cancel Culture, culture wars, the toppling of statues of those linked to the transatlantic slave trade, Trumpism, Fake News, the rise of the Far Right and Brexit have had an inevitable impact on our lives, our relationships and our work. Organisations and individuals have been forced to examine how our attitudes may have been shaped by racism, misogyny and unconscious bias. This may have always been the case but what is different now is that we are expected to act on what we have found. Those of us who have benefited from our class, colour, gender, sexuality, race and/or ability are being asked to check our privilege. White privilege allows white people such as me to move around the workplace relatively unmolested. (Except, as a woman, I am at risk of the things all women are, with the exception that I do not have to respond to colleagues' requests to touch my hair, as I have seen happen to black female colleagues.) However, at work I do not have to deal with the situation a black clinical friend described to me: he spoke of the often inevitable sharp intake of breath when he appears in the waiting room for the first time to collect a white family. I have found that families of colour seem never to be taken aback at *my* colour. The white clinician is perhaps the expected norm.

Statistics reflect that people of colour have been disproportionately affected by Covid with high numbers of deaths in that demographic. It may have caused some black staff members to be more fearful about going back into the workplace than others as their risk has been demonstrably higher. This has had to be taken into account when setting up rotas for clinical staff to be back in the clinic, face to face with colleagues and patients, albeit in masks. Supervisors have a role to play here in supporting those staff who may be worried about their risk and vulnerability. I was aware that some staff resented others who were allowed to work from home all the time and not pressured to go into the clinic (Morales and Ali 2021).

'When you're accustomed to privilege, equality feels like oppression.' It is not clear who first coined these words, but they reflect current schisms in society around entitlement and inequality. Entitlement connected to wealth, status, gender and class is being named and called out. All of this has, of course, affected relationships in the workplace between colleagues and with patients.

Silence, some would argue, is no longer an option. Power dynamics, and workplace and professional hierarchies, have become more visible in the context of these societal shockwaves. Race, class, gender, sexuality, age and ability are no longer 'add-ons' but the expectation is that these, the essence of a person, must be part of all clinical practice, including supervision. The workplace has changed and, as a result, the role and character of supervision has changed.

The socio-economic situation, the fallout from Covid, political upheaval and the targeting of migrants have led to dramatic and toxic splits and divisions within society and naturally, as a consequence, within some workplaces. Supervisees will be experiencing the effects of these, just as we supervisors are. I have found that it helps to bring the experiences of splits and divisions into supervision, where they can be heard and responded to. This is important because supervisees will be trying to manage the reactions of patients and colleagues to the situation. If the supervisee appears or sounds 'different', they carry an extra layer of stress and complexity as a result of stereotyping or racism that needs to be understood, addressed and in supervision.

Standing between accountability and support: the supervisor

Supervision, both clinical and managerial, is supposed to provide accountability to the employing organisation for both supervisee and supervisor. Supervision is part of quality control, it informs the appraisal process, and ideally monitors and builds the knowledge, skills and values of the supervisee. At its best, it is a developing process, not just a series of meetings, and should support, teach and help develop sound practice. The aim should be to improve the quality of clinical work, ensure safe practice and uphold the standards of service expected by the professional body and the employing organisation. Ultimately, it should ensure the provision of the best, safest and most effective treatment for children, teenagers and families. The supervisor derives their authority from the employing organisation as well as the professional organisation, but her primary responsibility is to the child. I want to look at how supervision and the role of the supervisor may have been affected by the constraints of the pandemic: online working, working from home, the reality of the serious illness and death of family, friends, colleagues and patients' relatives.

Formal and informal support structures

In my practice as a supervisor, I try to provide leadership, help clinicians organise and prioritise their work, find ways of speaking to managers if they are overburdened with cases and encourage them to work to their job plan. This is easier when they are in independent practice, but in the NHS or other organisations managers may be under pressure not to close waiting lists or turn referrals away. If NHS clinicians do not have support to protect their clinical thinking because of carrying too many complex cases, they can find that some service managers will assume clinical staff have endless time and resources to take on case after case. The workplace supervisor has a responsibility to their supervisees to protect this clinical work time and the space to process material and think. I have worked with clinicians who have been under such pressure in the NHS to see children that they have cancelled their supervision in order to take on another case.

The pandemic has limited daily, routine access to colleagues and senior professionals and, with high caseloads in a team, the work can become risky and unsafe. A major function of the multidisciplinary team is to provide a forum where risk is discussed and shared. Before the pandemic, face-to-face multidisciplinary team meetings could be extended on an impromptu basis or colleagues could meet in a small group afterwards to discuss ways of managing challenging cases. This opportunity for informal supervision has largely been lost with team contacts moving online. The loss of informal, on-the-hoof supervision, the corridor consultation, the coffee clinical conversation is likely to have led to a sense of isolation. Isolation can make work more stressful, lonelier, as it becomes harder for clinicians to share their thoughts and worries with colleagues and supervisors informally, be it popping into the office, having a walk around the block or over a cup of tea. Having to plan, book an online appointment with the supervisor rather than catching them in the kitchen or the corridor, can present supervisees with an obstacle, a boundary some may feel anxious about breaking.

Normal social contacts at work have largely disappeared as people work from home or attend work at the clinic on a rota basis, possibly not seeing some colleagues face to face for months on end. The loss of these informal, friendly, supportive interactions will leave us the poorer. What may once have seemed like trivial, superficial conversations about clothes, meals, holidays, family, cinema may now be accepted as serving an essential function for our well-being at work, oiling the wheels of teamwork, bonding teams together in laughter, and in hard times lifting spirits, putting work problems into perspective, lessening the stress and the pressure of long waiting lists, seriously ill patients and angry families. Clinicians used to be able to pop into the office of their supervisor in an unplanned way to run something by them. That can rarely happen now. If a clinician is at home and worried about a patient, they cannot, of course, talk to their own family members, but may not feel able to call their supervisor or manager without an online appointment. Instead of there being access to the team in the office at break times, where worries about patients can be aired perhaps on a daily basis, clinicians must often wait for their timetabled supervision session to discuss these in a more formal, less immediate, less raw way. It means they may be carrying more anxiety and worries than they might have done pre-pandemic. This is on top of managing their own and their families' mental and physical health. Staying in touch with colleagues has become very important, checking in with each other invaluable. Sharing anxieties about their own mental and physical health may not have always been part of team discussions but it strikes me as being an important aspect of staff support so that they can manage the extra stress of work during Covid. The frequent, daily, informal access, once taken for granted, should not be consigned to the past but it requires the will and energy to facilitate it.

Initially, there were, unsurprisingly, multiple logistical challenges to providing internet connection for employees so they could offer online therapy, work from home, attend meetings and have regular supervision. Although there have been advantages to clinicians working from home, there have been drawbacks, too. Working from home means no opportunities to socialise with colleagues as they would have had previously. This is such a vital part of the working day. Additionally, employees' ordinary physical activity, such as getting to work, walking from meeting to meeting, going up and down stairs will probably have decreased. When I was in Child and Adolescent Mental Health Services (CAMHS), I would walk about two miles a day just going from room to room, up and down corridors and stairs. Another disadvantage of working from home for some, is that it is hard to keep work life separate from home life. There is no interim period between leaving the clinic and arriving home during which they could de-stress, switch off. On top of this, it is likely that working from home has placed a strain on some couple/family relationships especially when children had to be home educated. Those with children have had to learn to juggle their usual responsibilities with childcare and home teaching and focus on work. Many will have been struggling in the same way as the parents of their patients: providing home schooling, unable to visit close relatives, fear for their families' health and well-being, cut off from elderly family in care homes or hospitals. All of these factors may well have equally been the case for some supervisors.

Supervision: adapting to the effects of the virus

Clinical supervision has always included a combination of the internal and the external. During the pandemic, the external has assumed greater importance, as we have all had to wrestle with the clinical parameters of working online and trying to protect the therapeutic space and continue to be reflective. However, physical constraints, public health concerns, including those around mental health, have forced us into new contexts in which supervision is now taking place and I have found that it has led to an expansion of my role of supervisor. I have sometimes become a sort of Occupational Health advisor, suggesting the clinician who works from home has a dedicated workspace, a desk or table and does not work from an armchair or their bed, sets up a routine, gets dressed, has breaks and lunch as they would at work. In my experience, checking on the supervisee's health has become an important part of supervision. I have found that their physical appearance, dress and manner might fluctuate between supervisions. I have tried to understand what working life is like for them, how they manage 'hybrid' working, working from home part of the week, being on a rota in other parts of the week to ensure safe distancing in the clinic and offices.

Teams may have lost close colleagues through poor health, family bereavement, even their own death. Colleagues will not have been allowed to attend the funeral of loved ones or to be with very ill or dying relatives. Yet, they have carried on working, providing the best service possible in the circumstances, treating children and families while shouldering the burden of their own trauma and distress.

Supervision for these clinicians may have assumed a much greater importance than before, providing a quiet space for reflection and support, offering some distance between patient and clinician through the perspective of the supervisor's view of a session.

Unfortunately, some highly valued colleagues have been lost to Brexit, returning to their home countries, perhaps after decades of working in the UK. Others may have fallen victim to the Home Office's 'Hostile Environment' exemplified by the treatment of the Windrush generation and their children, leading to the scandal of deportations (BBC News 2021). The hatred whipped up against refugees and asylum seekers has affected not only those who are 'othered' but also all those who work with colleagues and families from other countries. Colleagues whose accents, for example Polish or French, were never an issue in the past have become self-conscious about them, as I heard from one colleague. Their isolation from teams and colleagues might also exacerbate their sense of being apart, separate, being 'other'.

During any crisis, senior staff, in this case supervisors, support clinical staff by fostering a sense of containment, safety and leadership for supervisees. This may include managers and administrative staff. Pre-pandemic, they would ensure that they themselves had appropriate supervision, consultation and support. The Covid crisis has meant that supervisors themselves may require increased support for their own health, problems with being isolated, coping with their own family illnesses and deaths.

Even prior to Covid, good employers learned that supporting the physical and emotional well-being of their employees could help reduce stress, absenteeism and secondary trauma. During Covid, this has become even more significant. Setting realistic work goals for clinicians who may be under emotional pressure when working from home has become essential. I have heard from some clinicians that working from home has been easier than doing the daily commute and staying late in the clinic at the end of the day. The downside of this, though, is the loss of daily contact with others, of social interactions at work, which has been very hard for some clinicians.

The pandemic has reminded us that we are social animals. Like many others, I have longed for companionship and missed my relationships with family, friends and colleagues. I have even missed buildings and rooms, even when the journey to them once irritated or bored me. Perhaps we realise not only that we need each other, but that we enjoy each other. My own appreciation of others has certainly grown during this terrible period.

Child Psychotherapists, like other clinicians, have been left with the uncertainty of the safety of the workplace. Added to this are increased referrals, extreme pressures at work, little time to rest, to debrief with colleagues, and ongoing government cuts to services which have damaged staff morale. The anxiety around governmental incompetence, even indifference, has heightened people's fear of not being protected, and increased their uncertainty about the future. Delays in putting in place appropriate measures to protect the population and the failure to provide adequate personal protective equipment have been especially worrying and have led to a lack of containment, increased anxiety and heightened fear. It is not clear whether or not supervision has been able to provide adequate support for such deep-seated worries on top of very challenging clinical cases.

Safeguarding

Face-to-face psychotherapy, supervision and consultation have given way to online engagement, forcing change and flexibility in ways previously unthought of. The clinical space is no longer under the control of the therapist. The power has potentially shifted to the patients. They can decide how they want to engage: I work with young people who sometimes want the camera on, sometimes off, to be in the presence of their parents or alone. I have had dogs, cats, a bearded dragon, a toddler and a parrot in online sessions with patients. My own dog has proven to be particularly challenging and problematic for *me*, but it turns out he is a source of amusement and comfort for my patients, they tell me.

We have all been facing a frightening pandemic, but perhaps children have had a particularly difficult time. Along with isolation has come the fear and the reality of the death of older relatives and anxiety about their own future. Many teenagers, shut in their rooms, cut off physically from friends and normal activities, but with more intense online relationships, have come close to the edge of despair. They have been forced back into a position of dependence, which some may enjoy but others may experience as unbearable. The haphazard and confusing response of the Education Department around exams has been an unwelcome spanner in the works. Supervision has had to help clinicians think about how to address these practical and well-founded fears about the future in teenagers for whom unpredictability and uncertainty makes their lives feel unstable and fragile.

Some young people are able to speak in confidence in their bedroom, the parents' room or in some other space in or out of the home. However, others are clearly concerned about being overheard. This can lead to therapy being conducted while the young person is out walking in the park, at a friend's house or in the street. The supervisor who is forced to work this way with their own patients can help supervisees by providing resourcefulness, flexibility and support when therapy has to be delivered within these new physical freedoms and constraints. Regular, predictable contact with a trusted supervisor who can understand has been a source of reassurance for many clinicians. There is a normality and sense of safety in this relationship when it is not persecuting or unintentionally imbued with the supervisor's own anxiety.

Over the period of the pandemic, I suspect there has been a loss of confidence in leadership, a fear of not being kept safe by Government or employing organisations. In the past, this might have been mitigated by daily contact with colleagues experiencing similar worries. However, as a result of working from home, there has been a loss of impromptu, but significant, everyday, physical interaction with colleagues, discussing a difficult session over coffee in the kitchen where routine, informal debriefings would take place, possibly with cake and a hug proffered.

Supervision can sometimes be a source of intense anxiety in supervisees. This has had to be taken into account by the supervisor so that it does not aggravate anxieties about the pandemic. While some supervision can be experienced as persecuting, it is more often a source of relief, support, learning, challenge and development. However, the relationship between supervisor and supervisee has always been hierarchical, with a power imbalance, and there is a tension between the support and guidance provided and the element of assessment and judgement. This should lessen over time as the supervisee gains experience and confidence. Perhaps the experience of having a supervisor one trusts and from whom one derives containment, respect and validation during the time of Covid is one of the most important aspects of the clinician being able to survive a climate of physical illness, fear, paranoia and uncertainty.

Like other supervisors, I have had to be aware of my own need to manage fear, health anxiety and uncertainty and ensure these do not leak into the supervision space. At a time of enormous pressures on the NHS because of cuts and the pandemic, the organisation may have had to take greater account of the mental and physical health of its employees because of the enormous stress also placed on them.

Since the start of the pandemic, safeguarding has expanded beyond the usual physical and emotional safety to include environmental safety when working online (eye strain from too much screen time, for example), the wearing or not of masks, social distancing, effective ventilation. In some cases, it has been left to individuals to decide what is safe. It is possible that some patients and some professionals are still very anxious about the prospect of face-to-face working when it becomes more viable. What happens when the young person wants to meet face to face but the clinician is too anxious to do so? Where does responsibility for this lie? The supervisor needs to be able to offer guidance here, depending on the rules of the clinic in which the supervisee is working. There might be a case for a discussion about this between the supervisor and the clinic lead.

There have been concerns that substance abuse might be increasing because of the possibility of home deliveries of drugs and the more anonymous opportunity for shopping online for alcohol. A spotlight has fallen on some of the poorest families in the country with children going hungry and parents skipping meals in order to provide food for them. Fortunately, Marcus Rashford, a footballer who himself grew up in poverty, has highlighted the urgency for hungry children to be fed. To our shame, food banks have had to multiply across the country. Many poorer families have had no access to laptops, computers or phones so producing homework projects, submitting work, attending online lessons has not been possible for them. These are the children who could also not receive online therapy. Some children have experienced increased parental violence and parental substance abuse without the protective eye of teachers (The Guardian 2020).

An interesting, if voyeuristic, aspect of online working has been that it has allowed child psychotherapists into the homes of their young patients. Clinicians have seen their adolescent patients' bedrooms, a rare sight. They may also have been made aware of lack of space, privacy, furniture or the exact opposite. It certainly affected my own sense of the young people I work with to see their rooms behind them, and I think it probably affected the transference relationship for them to have an insight into my home and hear my heavily snoring dog, but I am still unsure in what way. My experience so far is that the sessions felt more open, more comfortable for some patients, maybe it has become a less one-sided power relationship. I would say that the same has happened with supervisees but that is only my opinion, I am not sure what they have felt about it.

Some supervisors have expressed their shock at the living conditions of some of their patients: their opulence or their deprivation. (Similarly, supervisees have had access to supervisors' rooms at home. Many of us will have been able to render their online backgrounds neutral and bland but not been able to block out the sound of neighbours, builders, dustmen, their own children – or in my case a noisy dog.)

Many families have had to try to provide a quiet, private, sound-proof space for their child to have their session. However, this has not always been possible and people have sometimes come in and out of the room where the session is being zoomed. Clinicians have had to provide the same for themselves when they are working clinically, needing to ensure their children do not walk in on a session or cause mayhem outside the door where they are working. Some group work has continued online but this has had its own challenges and limitations, many of which also apply to individual work and have been mentioned above.

Challenges to the traditional therapeutic frame

Clinicians, forced into working online with children/teenagers, have had to adapt to new, challenging ways of engaging their patients and maintaining therapeutic relationships. Patients and supervisees have become more aware of the technical abilities or anxieties of their therapists/supervisors. Some patients actually prefer working online and being able to choose whether or not to be on camera. There has been a shift in the power dynamic. Children can switch off the screen, bury themselves under their duvet, while the clinician can only look on. The clinical supervisor has had to find ways to help the management of these challenges to the therapeutic space. Children may want to see the clinician but not be seen themselves or vice versa. Some teenagers will want the camera on but will cover their faces. This is all new territory for child psychotherapists and their supervisors and there have been many discussions around how to manage the way young patients wish to have their sessions. It has been interesting to note how some adolescents reach a point where they want to be seen and will switch their camera on unexpectedly or the reverse might happen. These elements add an interesting dimension to psychotherapy and clinical supervision, as the camera, hidden or exposed faces, mark a change in the dynamic or in the transference relationship. Trying to make sense of these in supervision as part of process notes has become routine now. The clinical supervisor has had to help with the management of the challenges to the therapeutic space. They themselves have had to deal with similar fears and anxieties while continuing to provide training, containment and support along with fostering and monitoring the development of supervisees' psychoanalytic thinking.

An odd feature of online clinic meetings was described to me. Some staff attendees have turned off their cameras. This unusual behaviour was a challenge to the authority of the meeting's Chair and something of a disrespectful attitude to colleagues. I have not heard of this happening in supervision. I wonder how the Chair of such a meeting managed this novel, zoom-related problem.

Children who hate school and cannot manage groups, the journey to and from school and who endure bullying have found relief in being able to stay at home and have thrived. However, for some, cyber bullying has continued, in some cases even increased. The internet has boomed. Young people's lives have become even more dominated by platforms like Instagram, WhatsApp and TikTok. TikTok and YouTube have created a whole new raft of celebrities. For many of our young patients, YouTube videos are their main source of entertainment. It has been very impressive and gratifying that many young people attend their online therapy with the camera on and they focus for the duration of the session without simultaneously watching something on their phones. For those wanting to WhatsApp friends, play music, shout to siblings, talk to parents, watch something on their phone, at the same time as having their session, this has proven to be an extreme challenge to the therapist and has required practical support from the supervisor of the work. It's helpful if the supervisor, like me, has had similar difficulties with online patients, as it is important to help the supervisee in tangible ways yet also help them think about the meaning of multi-tasking in the session.

Nevertheless ...

In the midst of the chaos and fear, there is perhaps more, not less, need for good, regular, containing, thoughtful supervision. Supervisees still need to be helped to explore very difficult sessions when they might represent a transference object who is hated, feared, mistrusted. They may have to bear being experienced as an object who has murderous/abusive intentions. The virus is likely to make an appearance at some point in the work in one form or another. Supervisees may need help opening up about something in the patient's presentation that scares them, for example, fear of death, of emotional collapse, of perversion. They still need to bear being the object of passion or indifference. Supporting the thinking required to aid the supervisee to move down into the frightening world of their patient, their suicidal ideas, their hatred of the therapist, is an important and difficult task. Simultaneously helping the psychotherapist maintain their therapeutic stance and perspective in the throes of the emotional turmoil caused by the pandemic is also a huge challenge.

Despite the external risks and fears faced by clinicians, the responsibility of the supervisor is to help them continue the work in the face of psychosis, despair, narcissism, murderousness. What may be proving much more difficult in Covid times where there may be an atmosphere of paranoia may be how to understand and manage together patients who do not believe the virus really exists, who are aggressively against the vaccine and who may feel free to express racism, misogyny, homophobia, fear of refugees and of people who are 'different' in any way. The pressure on clinicians and supervisors around these issues has intensified in the context of the pandemic which may have aroused or increased psychosomatic disorders, feelings of paranoia, suicidal ideation.

Supervision has assumed a much more significant role during the pandemic. Thousands of deaths have been reported on a daily basis, numbers of cases shooting up all the time. The supervisor has needed to take account of the supervisee's own health, emotional well-being, home situation in a more overt way. Extended hours of screen exposure is known to cause fatigue, tiredness, headaches and sore eyes. Zoom fatigue has worn people down. In some cases, professionals sacrifice sleep in order to work at night or early in the morning while the rest of the house are asleep as these are hours when they can concentrate on work without interruption. All this has to be kept in mind when listening to clinical material being presented and robust, thoughtful supervision provided. There is no point in having a supervisor who listens patiently, nods, seems interested but can only offer, 'Yes, it's so hard working with this type of child/problem/family.'

The connection with their supervisor may well have become a bit of a lifeline to some clinicians who have lost valuable connections to their colleagues and workplace friends. It is a truism to say that companionship is essential for all of us, but it is especially important during times of crises, fear, trauma, uncertainty. At a time when we all have needed to be with family, friends and colleagues, we have been unable to do so, unable to give and receive support and comfort in the way we used to. The psychological impact on mental health clinicians has been enormous, perhaps especially for those clinicians who work with adolescents and who are also supporting their own teenagers at home. An adolescent's developmental need to separate and individuate has been compromised by having to stay at home and be dependent once more on parents for their daily needs. The supervisor might need to know about this in order to help the clinician manage their own feelings about their teenagers when working with adolescent patients, something which might have felt less necessary in earlier times.

Supervisors have had to draw on all their resources to help supervisees focus on the internal problems of their patients whilst acknowledging the ubiquitous presence of the uncertainty and threat of the external environment. The experience of the pandemic has been a universal one. Supervisors, supervisees and patients have all been caught in the same nightmare of losing people they love, fearing the loss of others, being trapped in isolation, experiencing the sometimes terrifying symptoms of Covid, unable to be with vulnerable friends and family. Who can ever forget the shocking reports of a child dying in hospital without his parents being able to hold him? Many care-home residents have died without family around them. These terrible, painful events may haunt us all even if we have not been directly affected.

The relationship between supervisor and supervisees, a central part of our work, has had to adapt to the strictures of the pandemic. Sharing a coffee, sitting across from each other, often set a comfortable context for the discussion of uncomfortable clinical work, burdened with projections from patients, families and the networks around the child. I have been aware that a more intense connection has developed with supervisees during the pandemic, their personal lives have become an important aspect of their capacity to provide psychotherapy in the way they were trained to. They, in turn, have had more intimate access to the home lives of their patients. Enforced flexibility, adaptation and dealing with online work with all of its quirkiness and unpredictability have changed our way of working clinically and discussing that work. When (and if) the pandemic ends, it will be interesting and helpful to take stock of what the Covid pandemic has introduced into the work of child psychotherapy and the supervision of these new ways of working.

References

BBC News (24 November 2021) Windrush generation: Who are they and why are they facing problems? https://www.bbc.co.uk/news/uk-43782241.

The Guardian (28 March 2020) Lockdowns around the world bring rise in domestic violence https://www.theguardian.com/society/2020/mar/28/lockdowns-world-rise-domestic-violence.

Mohdin, A (2022) Adultification. *The Guardian* 5 July.

Morales, D R and Ali, S N (2021) COVID-19 and disparities affecting ethnic minorities. *The Lancet 397* (*10286*): 1684–1685.

Shalhoub-Kervorkian, N (2019) *Incarcerated Childhood and the Politics of Unchilding* New York: Cambridge University Press.

Chapter 8

Supervising work with children and young people with a disability

Pamela Bartram

Children with a disability are, first of all, children. My thoughts about supervising work with these children are inevitably informed by my understanding of the wider principles of supervision. So, while I will reflect on some of the experiences and themes that recur, though probably not exclusively, where disability is part of the clinical picture, these are framed within the context of supervision in general. I will start with an example of one of the important ways in which I believe supervision works.

The patient listens in on the supervision?

At the end of a session with an academically high-achieving disabled adolescent patient I was left feeling frustrated. We had been working for a year or so, putting together a story about him which drew together his memories of childhood experience, the way it lives on in him in his everyday life and relationships and how at times we could see its impact on us 'right here right now'. We had thought about things from various points of view and, as a newcomer to psychotherapy, he found my thoughts in turn novel, enlightening, frightening, unbelievable, relieving, ridiculous and exciting.

Nevertheless, his emotional 'resting place' continued to be one of self-loathing which often found expression in self-harm.

Towards the end of that session, I found myself wondering what insight I had failed to bring. What understanding would bring about a change in his feelings about himself and in his worrying behaviour? In terms of the feeling quality of our relationship, I was dimly – preconsciously – aware of a certain 'scratchiness' in him, which I sensed served to keep me at an emotional distance, despite all the appearance – and not merely the appearance – of a good working alliance.

I took these impressions to supervision with a conscious hope that my supervisor would pick up on links I had failed to make. 'What am I missing? I asked.

My supervisor, however, picked up on the patient's intellectual defence. It seemed to have got into me. He and I were both hoping that finding out some

DOI: 10.4324/9781003297604-11

hitherto unrealised 'idea' about him would release him from his unhappiness. I saw that my search for more links and data was 'role responsive' (Sandler 1976) to his unconscious wish for an intellectual solution that would spare him emotional intimacy with me. My supervisor and I talked freely, and memories and associations came to mind. He had told me he would be worried to have a girlfriend in case she became too emotionally dependent on him. His fear of emotional dependency on me came into focus and I realised it stood in the way of a more radical shift in his well-being. My supervisor did not spell this out. This awareness came to mind in the course of a freely associative discussion with her about the patient and my experience of him.

The next session with the patient was two days later.

He began the session by saying, 'I'm exhausted by thinking.' A door opens.

How do we understand the process by which he arrived at this point in the work, showing his readiness to recognise the defensive nature of his thinking? The session which subsequently unfolded allowed us both to speak more openly about his need to keep me at an emotional distance and this, paradoxically, was the beginning of us coming closer. But that is another story.

How was my readiness to take my dilemma to my supervisor linked with her response to me and in turn with a new possibility opening up for the patient? Was the patient listening in on the supervision?

I suggest that unconsciously I already understood my patient's use of intellectual defence. In my search for more ideas, I mirrored it. I brought my understanding in an unconscious form to my supervisor who, in contact with me, brought it into my consciousness. I returned to my patient prepared to explore this and found that, in a parallel process, the patient had edged towards the same conclusion in the unconscious work he had done between the end of one session and the beginning of the next.

Supervision parallels the therapeutic process

Matryoshka dolls evoke something of the supervisor's function. The supervisor holds and understands the therapist in such a way as to support the therapist's ability to hold and understand the patient. It is likely that the supervisor has their own supervisor, who may in turn have their own supervisor, even if at some point this is an internalised supervisor rather than an external one. To understand the process of supervision of psychoanalytic work, which is my focus in this chapter, we may look at the ways in which it is similar to the process of psychoanalytic psychotherapy. 'The theories within psychoanalytic discourse have as much relation to psychoanalysis as a manual of sexual techniques has to the emotion of being in love.' (Symington 1986: 9). Theory and technique, of course, play a part but here I will focus on something else.

As I did in the example above, we may overestimate the importance of the concept, thought or idea and imagine that a large part of supervision involves the supervisor explaining the patient to the therapist. But in the same way that the therapist's task is not to explain the patient to himself, neither is it the supervisor's main job to explain the patient to the supervisee.

This is not to say that the supervisor brings nothing new to the table. She will say, 'This is how I see things.' But how she sees things will always be informed by her own emotional understanding of the supervisee and the patient's material as mediated through the vision and response of the therapist in supervision.

Supervising work with disabled children, adolescents and their families

I now turn to the question of specific themes or experiences which may characterise work where a disability is part of the clinical picture and which, therefore, are likely to emerge as live issues in supervision.

The messiness of the work

When people bring new cases to me for supervision, initially it can be as if a whirlwind or flood has entered the room. The supervisee conveys a sense to me of a great spreading mess of ... something ... elemental ... thoughts, feelings, experiences, unprocessed and uncontained.

Children with a disability are more psychologically vulnerable than their 'mainstream' peers. An accumulation of experiences contributes to this. They may have: limited access to the binding power of language and thinking; a daily experience of themselves as looking and sounding unattractively and unacceptably different from their peers; experience of early traumatic separations and intrusions; the experience of parental grief and depression; been deprived of opportunities to play instead of attending remedial therapy/work sessions; regular encounters with environmental factors that lead to their exclusion or rejection from social settings; limited opportunities for peer relationships; repeated exposure to the emotional experience of social rejection and revilement.

All of these militate against ego development and may leave the patient at the mercy of unbound elemental forces, including psychic pain, rage and grief.

The therapist who struggles to tolerate chaotic mess may find themselves severely tested.

Case
A trainee brought to me a case from his NHS work for an initial supervision session. The child had various diagnoses and the network was complex and hard to hold in mind. There were financial and emotional problems in the family. I quickly felt overwhelmed by the raw material and, although the trainee did not say that he felt overwhelmed by the case, I thought that at least some of my response was a communication from him.

After the trainee left, two thoughts preoccupied me. Can psychotherapy contain this amount of chaos, dysfunction and disturbance? The second was to doubt my own ability and experience to hold the case. I had not worked in the NHS for some years and perhaps I was not up to this level of complexity. I consulted first with my own internal supervisor and when she proved less than helpful, with my external one.

I started supervising the case on a regular basis and the child went on to make good progress and good use of the therapy.

Sometimes the chaotic nature of the child's communications takes time to emerge and only does so once they have a sense that their therapist will be able to manage it. Valerie Sinason talked about 'the handicapped smile' of the patient who protects the world from knowing the patient's true feelings about themselves and others by presenting an obliging and non-threatening smile (Sinason 2010: 124–125). Moving beyond this can be an essential part of the therapy.

Case
Eight-year-old Lara had a diagnosis of developmental delay. She was referred to psychotherapy because of her physical and verbal aggression to her parents. She was described as having violent rages and had self-harmed in a way deemed unusual and worrying for a child of her age.

Lara initially presented as chatty and smiley but in time she started to create floods and mess with the water and sand tray. She communicated an experience of feeling overflowing and flooded. The therapist often felt angry about the mess created in the room and brought this anger to supervision.

I, in turn, felt flooded by the therapist's distressed and angry feelings, but I was also able to remind her that her patient might have too much ego strength invested in repressing powerful and chaotic feelings. If they could be released and communicated to her therapist, more of her ego strength would be available for other tasks.

I think the trainee felt that I stood with her in the face of the child's messy and sometimes destructive behaviour, and this allowed her to tolerate it and communicate with Lara.

In time, Lara played in ways more typical of a latency child, setting up the doll's house and dolls, playing games with rules, and she was more able to express her thoughts and feelings in words. The storm of her feelings had been weathered and this allowed her to bring other aspects of herself to the fore.

The projection of disability

We all live with the tension between working within our limitations, on the one hand, and, on the other, striving to expand the scope of our ability.

I have already mentioned the experience of feeling not up to the job, or disabled, a feeling which may lodge in the supervisee and in the supervisor too. Unsurprisingly, this is another common experience in working with disabled children.

Case
James had cerebral palsy. He looked and sounded different from his peers. He spent much of his time in therapy tying his therapist up with string and Sellotape and sometimes this felt almost unbearable for her. She felt a sense of dread and fear and had to judge carefully both how much she could tolerate and how useful it was for him to give her this experience. Sometimes she felt unable to make this decision, as if she had lost her autonomy. She brought all these states of mind to supervision which offered a space away from the immediacy of the pro-jections in which she could digest the experience of being stuck and immobile.

Disabled children and adults often look and sound very different from 'mainstream people', and often society imposes further limitations on them by limiting their opportunities to take part in the activities of ordinary life. How can an autistic child manage the sensory and social experience of a cinema? How does a mother take her wheelchair-user child on a tube journey? How hard do the parents of an unruly autistic boy have to fight for a Blue Badge parking permit? How does an adolescent with Down's syndrome lose their virginity in a consensual sexual relationship? It is not surprising, therefore, that work with disabled children and adolescents throws up a multilayered experience of being bound by limitations, some imposed by the disability itself, others by defences against the pain of feeling lesser than others and others by the environment's response to disability.

Both the therapist and the supervisor will need to be able to tolerate this experience.

A disabled network

It is common to find that, unlike their mainstream peers, a child with a disability has several professionals actively involved in their health and education. This situ-ation offers the possibility of a network around the child, which may function more or less well.

Sometimes the experience of disability is expressed not primarily in a sense of impotence or helplessness, as in the case of James above, but in a disorder of communication. In both cases, the network may be challenged by such projections and find itself disabled but unaware of this. When such projections remain uncon-scious, they are likely to give rise to a network that does not function effectively.

Like the individuals within it, the network is susceptible to the excessive use of defences when confronted with something that cannot be 'fixed', even though other things could be significantly improved and others repaired.

Sometimes failing to put the pieces together is a way of avoiding the distress involved in seeing the whole picture.

Case

A child psychotherapist was working with Luke, a ten-year-old boy with complex needs. He had a school place but was not attending. Luke had a serious physical health illness, as well as having been diagnosed with autism spectrum disorder (ASD). Issues in the wider family, some to do with his difficulties and others less so, militated against an ordinary and age-appropriate level of separation between the child and his single mother. Supported by her supervisor, the psychotherapist set about familiarising herself with the network with a view to getting involved. She found that the 'network' was not functioning. Some parts of it acted autonomously and others were entirely moribund.

Supervision offered a useful space in which the child psychotherapist could express her frustration, anger and distress about the lack of a concerted effort to improve life for the child. At times she felt that she alone in the 'network' could imagine a better life for him, while others seemed to have given up hope. A key role of the supervisor was to be in touch with the psychotherapist's hopefulness and drive, her wish to join things up and look at the whole picture, however distressing. Supervision helped the therapist to feel she was not mad to imagine a more fulfilled life for Luke.

Separation difficulties

When a baby is born with a disability, or later discovered to be disabled, the ordinary, good-enough parents recognise that their child is likely to need more support and supporting agencies in their life than does the average mainstream child. Parents may find themselves working with several professionals who advise on what input their child needs, such as speech and language therapists, physiotherapists, occupational therapists, paediatricians, as well as psychological therapists. In the early days of assessment and diagnosis, parents may feel they have to gear themselves up to attend many appointments, carry out therapy exercises at home, giving time and energy to doing their best for their baby or child. I have written elsewhere about how this can impact on family life, especially on the parents' partnership and on siblings (Bartram 2007: Chapters 8 and 9).

Trauma may play an important part in the family's history: a traumatic birth, diagnosis or medical interventions, any of which may complicate the process of separation.

Parents are confronted by the fact that their child's development is delayed in comparison to that of their peers and worry about how their child will survive in the world without all the additional care and attention the parents are providing. Ultimately this expresses itself in the question 'Who will look after them when we are dead?'

These worries can make the process of psychological and physical separation more difficult. Ordinary developmental stages, such as weaning, sleeping alone, starting nursery or school, having play dates and the emergence of adolescent sexuality, may be fraught with additional emotional difficulties for parents and child.

Setting boundaries and saying 'no', which are essential for psychological development, may be difficult for parents of disabled children because it feels cruel to deprive them of short-term pleasure.

The psychotherapist may need to be prepared for parents to find it difficult to allow their child a separate space in psychotherapy, sometimes at some level feeling guilty for what a relief it is to let them go. It may be necessary to work with parent (or parents) and child to help them to separate. The psychotherapist may need to be sensitive to the life-and-death fears around separation which children and parents may share.

The supervisor can support the therapist to tolerate difficulties with separation and sometimes to sustain a closer relationship with the child's parents than might usually be the case.

Case

An 11-year-old boy with a pervasive developmental disorder repeatedly left the consulting room, ostensibly to look for his parents who were being seen in another consulting room. The therapist allowed this, feeling that the child needed to reassure himself that his parents were available. The child still slept in his parents' bed at night and, after a period of thoughtful tolerance, the supervisor began to feel a growing sense of irritation that the child intruded upon his parents' session.

The supervisor and supervisee talked through the situation. The supervisor contained her sense of irritation but pointed out the intrusive nature of the child's behaviour, while also acknowledging the anxiety that underlay it.

The supervisor suggested to the supervisee the importance of preventing the child from leaving the room by, for example, placing his chair against the door. This was not to be punitive but to create an opportunity for the therapist to experience more directly the child's underlying distress and need for control.

The supervisee appeared to see the point and even to agree, but week after week, continued to follow the child through the clinic to the room where his parents were being seen.

The therapist could not bring himself to follow the supervisor's advice, as he felt it was cruel to prevent the child from checking up on his parents.

(Incidentally, mother felt it was cruel to exclude the child from the parental bed, even though father was quite sick of the family's sleeping arrangements.)

Supervisor and supervisee tolerated this situation for some time. Then came a point when something shifted in the supervisee and he took a firmer stand, which proved helpful to the child both in terms of using his psychotherapy and in the sleeping arrangements at home. No doubt there had to be a deep emotional shift in the therapist for him to be able to use the technical advice of the supervisor. When he could do so, the child started to sleep in his own bed.

It was no good for the supervisor to think critically, 'Why is this supervisee not following my advice?' She respected his need to 'know' deeply that a change of technique was needed. The supervisor was aware that there were almost certainly unconscious factors in the supervisee to do with his own unresolved experience of separation and loss, though she did not explore these with the supervisee, as this would be beyond her remit.

The supervisor will at times bring in advice on technique and this can contribute to the supervisee's experience. However, I suggest that without the context of Neville Symington's 'intersubjective emotional understanding' (1986: 324) or Kenneth Wright's 'symbolic location' (2009: 35) it cannot provide what is needed.

Because we offer advice on technique, we cannot assume it can be used by the supervisee. The supervisor who tells her supervisee *what to say* to the patient is misguided. The supervisor is no more in a position to sort out the supervisee by telling her what to do than is the therapist in a position to sort out the patient by the same method. How much more quickly would our work be completed if only difficulties could be resolved that way!

It is important for the supervisor to help the therapist to occupy a place where she can make an authentic emotional connection with her patient. Once that is established, insights and their expression in words will follow.

Melancholia and the superego

I have written elsewhere about the harsh superego that may mobilise in cases where disability is a factor (Bartram 2013) and other child psychotherapists have written about the same phenomenon (Miller 2002).

In 'Mourning and melancholia', Freud says that in melancholia, we find low self-regard, 'self-reproaches, self-revilings' and 'delusional expectation of punishment' (Freud [1915]1917: 244).

Parents may blame themselves, consciously or unconsciously, and feel they deserve to be punished for their child's disability. They may drive themselves to exhaustion by researching treatments, attending appointments, doing programmes of exercises with their child and neglect their own need for space and recreation, and indeed their child's need for the same.

Children and adolescents may hate themselves for their 'stupidity', as if having a learning disability is a moral failure.

Deborah Marks indicates that these punishing states of mind may be acted out within the professional network as well as within the individual and the family unit. Quoting Mason, she says: 'Other children play but you do therapy. Other children develop but you are "trained". Almost every activity of daily living can take on the dimension of trying to make you less like yourself ...' (Marks 1999: 69).

These practices and the state of mind from which they emanate interfere with the experience of 'going-on-being' (Winnicott 1960) which is necessary for health. Marks continues:

Thus the kind of interdisciplinary practices enacted upon the physically disabled person (or the person with learning difficulties ...) are more intensive than those imposed upon the "normal" ... The experience, particularly for the infant or young child, of having things constantly *done to them* ... can be disruptive to their "continuity of being" and therefore traumatic.

(Marks 1999: 69, emphasis in original)

The supervisor, who is in a position of power in relation to the therapist, may find herself susceptible to offering a home to harshly critical states of mind which have an intrapsychic counterpart.

The therapist may struggle with judgemental thoughts about his own work, its lack of efficacy or slow progress.

Symington commented on the 'very powerful group superego operative within the psychoanalytic community' (Symington 1986: 327). Some authors infer from clinical experience that parents feel horror, shock and disappointment when looking at their disabled baby and that the baby internalises this and grows up feeling 'unworthy of love and deserving of rejection' (e.g., Emanuel 1997: 280 and Miller 2002: 30). I think it is important not to generalise from inferences about children in psychotherapy to statements about the parents of disabled children in general, many of whom provide lifelong loving care for their babies and children, wrestling humanely and even heroically with emotional pain and practical challenges.

Freud and man's soul

God, grant me the serenity to accept the things I cannot change,
courage to change the things I can,
and wisdom to know the difference.

(The Serenity Prayer)[1]

Contact with disability reminds us of our vulnerabilities, challenges our omnipotence and narcissism and faces us with our common humanity. Where we cannot tolerate our own vulnerabilities, we may project them into others, distance ourselves from them, hate them 'over there' and exclude the disabled (and other groups) from mainstream society by, for example, making much of it inaccessible to them.

In work with disabled children there is a danger of 'taking the part for the whole' or attributing every so-called 'problematic' characteristic of the child to the condition or disability with which they have been diagnosed.

Bettelheim reminds us that Freud uses the term 'soul' for what we are treating and that, 'By evoking the image of the soul and all its associations, Freud is emphasising our common humanity' (Bettelheim 1985: 71).

It worries me to hear generalisations about 'people with Down's syndrome' or 'people with autism'. In psychotherapy we work with the whole human being: their

innate endowment, the psyche-soma; the impact of life experience and developmental stage. They all contribute to the patient's experience of themselves and
others, to the totality of their consciousness and unconsciousness. I have often
noticed that notes on sessions with disabled children are rarely distinguishable from
any other notes, because the therapist is not recording data about a disability but
about a person.

Case

A three-year-old child with Down's syndrome had been introduced to her baby
brother for the first time. In the joint mother-child therapy session, she became
cross, threw her toys around and 'forgot' her toilet training progress. Her mum
attributed these developments to her Down's syndrome and her 'inability to
understand' what was happening in the family. My child psychotherapy supervisee believed that the little girl understood perfectly well what was going on
in the family. Whatever her cognitive impairment, she did know that a baby
brother was bringing big changes, and, from her point of view, not necessarily
for the better!

I agreed with my supervisee. We both felt it was an important part of the work to
try to help her parents to think about the emotional life of their daughter instead
of attributing her responses solely to the condition she had been diagnosed with.

Case

A therapist started some parent work with the parents of a teenage boy with ASD.
With the onset of adolescence, he had become increasingly rigid and controlling at home and family life was shrinking to fit in with his, at times, quite cruel
demands. The therapist tried to think with the parents about what aspects of his
feelings and behaviour might be amenable to change through emotional understanding. These parents had spent his early years implementing a rigid system of
behavioural intervention, and for them everything their son did was an expression of his autism and could not be helped. They saw him as a victim of his
condition. The idea of adolescence as a time when he might feel the need to
reinforce his defences in the face of unstoppable changes in his psyche-soma did
not make sense to them. The therapist and the parents were speaking two different
languages.

The therapist felt she could not breach the 'language barrier' and the supervisor
supported her to end the work, rather than take the parents into ongoing psychoanalytically informed parent work.

Fortunately, psychoanalytic psychotherapists working in the Independent tradition are unlikely either to confuse the child with their diagnosis or to forget how
the child's developmental stage impacts on and is impacted by other areas of their
experience. Psychotherapists' experience as patients in analysis helps them, we
hope, to know and tolerate their own flawed, imperfect selves.

Concluding thoughts: psychotherapy, mourning and hope

Winnicott tells us:

> Psychotherapy is not making clever and apt interpretations; by and large it is a long-term giving the patient back what the patient brings. It is a complex derivative of the face that reflects what is there to be seen. I like to think of my work this way, and to think that if I do this well enough the patient will find his or her own self, and will be able to exist and feel real. Feeling real is more than existing; it is finding a way to exist as oneself, and to relate to objects as oneself, and to have a self into which to retreat for relaxation.
>
> (Winnicott 1971: 137)

As psychotherapists, we spend much of our time in contact with the patient's defences against grief: overactivity, self-revilement, grandiosity, denial and more. Yet at the same time, we are aware, sometimes less sometimes more acutely, of the pain against which those defences have been rallied. Healing takes place when the wound is known, its pain shared, and when mourning eclipses melancholia. This allows the patient to find, in Winnicott's words, 'his or her own self', to 'feel real', to hope and to search out and grasp life.

It would be misguided to think that work with children and adolescents with a disability is all about mourning, although of course the themes of loss, what might have been and what never will be, are always part of the picture. But is this not true for all patients in psychotherapy, indeed for us all?

Perhaps the need to mourn is particularly important for parents of children with a disability, so that in our work with them we must open ourselves to the intense sadness they sometimes feel, to their 'chronic sorrow' and 'cyclic mourning' (Davis 1987: 352).

In my experience, feelings of grief are more available to consciousness in adolescents and adult patients than in younger patients: the 15-year-old autistic boy feels trapped in his family, describes himself as 'useless', has no friend and no hope of one; the middle-aged woman with Down's syndrome, who becomes an aunt for the second time, weeps when she tells her therapist she will never be a mother; the 18-year-old girl with an intellectual disability sobs in the consulting room after her first week at college, where she was called 'spaz' by the 'cool kids'.

Are these depths of sorrow deeper than the sorrow of other 'non-disabled' people? I don't know how to measure sorrow.

Supervision supports the psychotherapist to stay in touch with the patient and all they bring. To reduce the work to dealing with pain and sorrow would be to miss the powerful presence of humour, celebration, gratitude and hope that enliven both the work itself and the supervisor's engagement with it.

If the therapist's job is to help the patient to 'find his or her own self', to 'feel real' and to 'have a self into which to retreat for relaxation', we may say that the supervisor's job is not dissimilar. Supervision supports the 'common humanity' of psychotherapist and patient, which is the foundation for change.

Note

1   Extract from prayer attributed to American theologian Reinhold Niebuhr (1892–1971)

References

Bartram, P (2007) *Understanding Your Young Child with Special Needs* The Tavistock Clinic London: Jessica Kingsley.

Bartram, P (2013) Melancholia, mourning, love. *British Journal of Psychotherapy 29* (*2*): 168–181.

Bettelheim, B (1985) *Freud and Man's Soul* London: Fontana.

Davis, B (1987) Disability and grief. *Social Casework 68*: 352–357.

Emanuel, L (1997) Facing the damage together. *Journal of Child Psychotherapy 23* (*2*): 279–302.

Freud, S ([1915]1917) Mourning and melancholia *SE XIV* London: Hogarth Press.

Marks, D (1999) *Disability: Controversial Debates and Psychosocial Perspectives* London: Routledge.

Miller, L (2002) Adolescents with learning disabilities: psychic structures that are not conducive to learning. *Journal of Child Psychotherapy 28* (*1*): 29–39.

Sandler, J (1976) Countertransference and role responsiveness. *International Review of Psychoanalysis 3*: 43–47.

Sinason, V (2010) *Mental Handicap and the Human Condition* London: Free Association Books.

Symington, N (1986) *The Analytic Experience* London: Free Association Books.

Winnicott, D W (1960) The theory of the parent-infant relationship. *The International. Journal of Psycho-Analysis 41*: 585–595.

Winnicott, D W ([1971]1974) Mirror-role of mother and family. In *Playing and Reality* London: Pelican.

Wright, K (2009) *Mirroring and Attunement: Self-realisation in Psychoanalysis and Art* Hove: Routledge.

Chapter 9

Enhancing practice

Consultation to a therapeutic fostering agency

Iris Gibbs

Introduction

The chapters in this book are mainly about supervision, whilst the focus in this chapter is on consultation, as offered by a child and adolescent psychotherapist. The context for the consultation is a private organisation that provides therapeutic foster care for children and young people considered to be at physical and/or emotional risk and removed from their birth families. In recent years the organisation has also taken in several unaccompanied minors seeking asylum in the UK. As they are younger than 18, they come under the umbrella of social service departments and have been placed in either foster care or a residential facility. Many arrive with psychological problems and other health and educational needs resulting from leaving their family and country as well as experiencing further trauma in the search for asylum. Digidiki and Bhabha (2017) write that their experience of the immigration system can also compound the existing trauma, as the young people often have to recount harrowing experiences in great detail to justify their asylum claim. Crawley (2007) writes about the long wait for decisions on asylum claims and the impact this has on the capacity of these young people to mourn what has been lost from their childhood and adolescence. Most significantly, it is seen as interfering with their ability to develop a secure sense of identity in the new country. Akhtar (1999) writes of the totality of the unaccompanied minors' experience as one that recalls too many 'little deaths' with repeated separations, losses and cultural dislocation, resulting in the primitive anxiety of annihilation.

Throughout this chapter, I reflect on the ways my training in child and adolescent psychotherapy has enabled me to fulfil my role as consultant to a team who look after the needs of these vulnerable children and young people. In a changing world where, increasingly, much is expected of this profession, the ability to adapt the psychotherapy training to meet the needs of a diverse population will be crucial to its survival. Two of the areas in which trained psychotherapists can be influential are supervision and consultation. These terms are often used interchangeably, but there are differences as well as similarities, which I will address. In describing the consultation process. I will draw on my own experience, including illustrative case

DOI: 10.4324/9781003297604-12

material, as well as relevant literature in the field. Finally, I will consider briefly the question of research-based evidence on the effectiveness of consultation.

The team

The team I consult to includes two managers, who oversee the work of the team as a whole, five trained social workers, who supervise the foster carers, and an educa-tion specialist, who liaises with schools and colleges. The role of the education spe-cialist is hugely important as many of the children and young people placed have experienced disruptions in their learning due to frequent changes of placement and school. It is not unusual for some to come to the organisation without the basic academic skills appropriate to their ages. When this is compounded by behavioural and emotional difficulties many find it difficult to manage in a mainstream school setting and are allocated other education provision. I have been consultant to the team for ten years, but my contact with the organisation goes back more than 20, in a variety of roles – providing psychotherapy to children and young people, super-vising trainees, facilitating individual and reflective group sessions with foster car-ers, teaching theory and chairing management discussions on race and cultural issues. This wide experience has given me much insight in how the organisation functions, and it was a privilege to be asked to be a consultant to the team which is based in an ethnically diverse area of London. The team, foster carers and children in placement reflect the diverse make-up of the local area, as well as the children and young people who are accommodated from other parts of London and further afield.

It is a rewarding experience to consult to an organisation that seeks to understand and address challenges and to work diligently to ensure that the children and young people are not further disadvantaged by being in care. The team also works closely with social services departments who retain overall responsibility for the children and young people. In common with other childcare agencies, the organisation is regularly inspected by Ofsted (the Office for Standards in Education, Children's Services and Skills) and is consistently rated as outstanding. As consultant, I can also be asked to comment on the organisation's ability to meet the complex needs of the children and young people. Whilst there have been changes in management over time, the organisation has remained committed to using all available resources to train and equip both the supervising team and foster carers to meet the needs of the children and young people, including the use of external professional services.

The child psychotherapist as consultant

In seeking consultation from a child and adolescent psychotherapist, the managers wanted to ensure that the staff group was well informed about child development and how this can be derailed by adverse experiences. Lanyado (2009) draws atten-tion to the long tradition within child psychotherapy of offering clinical supervi-sion and consultation to the childcare professions. Sprince (2002) writes that it is also important for the professionals to actively work on understanding themselves and their processes of relating. It is an area that the psychoanalytically informed consultant will be concerned with, as it encourages the carers to do the same, which in turn will have a positive impact on those in placement. The ability to be in touch with feelings, to have them contained and put into words when possible, is particularly important for those children and young people who would have had problems sharing deeper feelings with others. In the case of unaccompanied minors, Melzak, McLoughlin and Watt (2018) suggest such feelings may include helplessness and anxieties about abandonment, rage at sequential injustice and sadness relating to massive loss, shame and guilt.

Hunter-Smallbone (2009) views the training of child psychotherapists as well suited to the careful weaving together of these children's shattered emotional lives. Child psychotherapists, she argues, are trained to bear witness, to emotionally contain and to reflect on the despair and extreme, unresolved states of mourning often experienced by foster children. Melzak et al. (2018) also point out that it often falls to the child psychotherapist to communicate vulnerabilities in children to other colleagues in the caring professions. Both Gibbs (2006) and Robinson, Luyten and Midgley (2017) note the particular contribution child psychotherapists can make in staff and network meetings, where the focus is often on external behaviour rather than the children's internal worlds and unconscious ways of relating. Psychotherapists are also seen as holding a key position in helping the network to think about processes that can occur in systems around distressed and disturbed children and young people.

My consultant role draws heavily on insights gained from my training in the Independent psychoanalytic tradition, an approach that introduces the therapist to all the major theoretical schools of thought. In my role consulting to the team, I found Bion's concept of containment (1962) and Winnicott's holding environment (1965) particularly helpful. The concepts were originally used in relation to infants and their caregivers but have subsequently been applied to a range of relationships and settings, including social work and consultancy. Ogden (2004) notes that the terms are often linked together and makes the following distinction. He defines Winnicott's holding as primarily concerned with being and its relationship to time, whilst Bion's model is centrally concerned with the processing of thoughts derived from lived experience. Like Ogden, I do not see the concepts as standing in opposition to each other, rather as two vantage points from which to view an emotional experience.

For the purpose of this chapter, containment involves receiving the emotional communication from team members, processing this and communicating it back with understanding and recognition. It can be thought of as providing a space for thinking in circumstances that may lead the team to do the opposite and involves the consultant using her counter-transference as a source of information that helps the team with their management of tasks (Douglas 2007). In terms of the holding environment, I have found Kahn's (2001) views particularly helpful in relation to my consultation work. Whilst less intensive than Winnicott's holding of a mother, or that of an analyst, Kahn suggests that a holding environment offers a reasonably safe place in which people may examine and express their experiences. However, he acknowledges that it is a different matter to create such environments for adults whose work is fast paced, whose time and energies are scarce and who are in organisations often marked by frequent turnovers and other major transitions. Nonetheless, for Kahn, it is in precisely these circumstances that the holding environment is considered most useful for working through potentially debilitating anxieties. Ruch's holistic model (2011) brings together the emotional, organisational and epistemological elements of containment and holding, which I also found helpful. Applying this to my work, consultation becomes a system of support or organisational holding in which a shared understanding of the tasks can be considered and where different interpretations of the task can be responded to thoughtfully.

A definition of consultation

Jacquelyn Kirby in her *New Perspective Consultation & Supervision* blog (2022) defines consultation as a cooperative relationship, unlike supervision which tends to be more hierarchical. However, both function to encourage more efficient, independent, self-aware workers, who are able to recognise strengths and areas needing to be further developed. In both cases, the therapist needs to be aware of covert feelings, splits, defences, group dynamics and other interpersonal processes that could hinder progress.

Schein (1990) proposes three models of consultation, which I have found helpful in determining the approach I use. The author distinguishes between the 'expert', 'playing the doctor' and 'process' models. The process consultation model is based on a set of assumptions that Schein argues are better suited to the human systems with which we typically deal. Firstly, it assumes that clients often seek help when they do not know what the problem is and what kinds of help are available. Secondly, most clients benefit from participation in the diagnostic process since, so often, they are part of the problem and may need help in recognising this. Thirdly, only clients know what form of remedial intervention will really work, because they know what will fit their personalities, their group and organisational culture. Lastly, Schein puts forward the idea that clients have 'constructive intent' and will therefore benefit from the process of learning that enables them to manage similar situations in the future.

Gabbard (2000) further warns that consultants should avoid a critical or disapproving stance, lest this interfere with the consultee's capacity to share openly details of the problem. The consultant will also need to be aware of their own biases and be able to develop a mutual enquiry process that not only creates a shared sense of responsibility for figuring out what is wrong and how to fix it, but also enables the consultant to pass on some of their diagnostic and intervention skills. Schein refers to this as 'helping the client learn how to learn' (1990: 60) The consultant process model does not rule out an expert role if this is indicated, but Schein suggests that it should come only after a spirit of genuine exploratory enquiry has been established and insights gained, so as to ensure that the consultee continues to own both the problem and the solution. He also cautions against falling in with the popular view of consultants by adopting the doctor role and responding to the invitation to investigate, interview, make a diagnosis and suggest a cure. This presupposes that the client has correctly identified where the 'sickness' lies, has revealed the information necessary for a good diagnosis, will do what the doctor recommends and will remain healthy when the doctor leaves. This model for Schein goes awry, as one or more of the above assumptions often cannot be met.

I have quoted extensively from Schein as his process consultation model is the one that I use with the team. It is also important to bear in mind that, in offering this consultation, there can be at least three sets of people to consider simultaneously – the supervising team, the foster families and the stakeholders. Therefore, though psychoanalytically informed, interventions need to be systemic, as they must be considered in terms of the consequences to other parts of the system, even if as consultant I am not directly involved at all levels. Based on this premise, the tools, methods and theories I select have to be appropriate to the information provided and facilitate an intervention that will address concerns within the organisational context. Kahn (2001) helpfully recommends that consultants should stay within given roles, tasks and boundaries. This is in acknowledgement of the fact that mature dependency also entails a move towards independence (Winnicott 1965). Otherwise, there is a risk that those being held may become dependent, and those doing the holding may become overly controlling and lose sight of the task of developing capacities, one of the essential roles of consultancy.

My consultancy work varies according to the needs of the team, but always remains within my areas of competence. I can be part of the thinking about matching a child or young person with a carer. Whilst differences in terms of race, ethnicity and gender are all part of the thinking, the resources in the carer to meet wider needs are given equal consideration. Thinking about the child's history in terms of what is, or is not, known is important, as this can have a bearing on the success or failure of a placement. It is worth noting that the children and young people who cope better in placements tend to be those who have an ongoing relationship with a social worker or other trusted adult who knows their history. In placing children and young people, consideration is also given to the level of contact with parents and other family members, as there can be conflicts which may undermine the placement. Unfortunately, not all placements succeed and the thinking in these situations is then about how to achieve as good an ending as possible. This is important in attempting to break the seesaw cycle of fleeting contacts followed by repeated abandonments experienced by some children and young people.

Lanyado (2017) reminds us that many of these children and young people find it difficult to put down roots in the potentially nurturing soil of new relationships. Because of their traumatic past experiences, they tend to erect barriers to protect themselves from further pain. Much organisational effort goes into training and preparing carers, but for some children and young people, particularly those who are placed as adolescents, the intimacy of a foster family can go against the thrust of adolescent development. For such children the relative autonomy of a residential placement is more attractive. Though a move is ultimately the responsibility of the child's allocated local authority social worker, I can be part of this thinking, i.e., how and where the young person's physical and psychological needs will be best met and in what timescale. This has implications, not just for their period in care, but in preparing them for life beyond the care system.

Supporting foster carers

In a previous publication I described how the foster carer's task, once considered so natural as to require little in the way of training or special expertise, has had to be re-evaluated because of the complex needs of the children in their charge (Gibbs 2006). Ironside sums up the expectations now placed on foster carers:

> To maintain a reflective capacity and to be able to be close to the child, to experience the often traumatic, emotional nature of such a relationship, to bear witness and to contain the child's states of despair, yet to be distant enough not to be overwhelmed by it.
>
> Ironside (2009: 329)

Much stress is placed on the need for adequate training, and this is given high priority in the organisation I consult to. Wheal (1999) also suggests that in addition to training, foster carers need to be professionally supported to meet demands. This need is acknowledged by the organisation, and provision is made for private therapeutic support if needed. Carers also attend a monthly reflective group, which I facilitate and, when needed, I meet with carers individually or jointly with their supervising social workers, as illustrated in the following vignettes.

Vignette 1

Vicky was 15 and had been in local authority care since the age of eight, after being removed from the care of her mentally ill mother. Although the possibility of adoption was raised, the thinking at the time was that she might be returned to her family following a period in care. This did not happen and she was placed permanently with foster carers. Much of Vicky's early placement difficulties revolved around the sporadic contact between her and her birth mother. Despite this, and because of her young age, Vicky thrived with the care and consistency provided by her placement and individual therapeutic support. This changed as Vicky entered adolescence, which also coincided with her ending therapy. By the age of 15 she was staying out all night and engaging in behaviours that put her at risk of physical and sexual harm. This caused severe disruption to the lives of the carers and others in the household. There followed much inter-agency support, in an attempt to manage the situation, but it took its toll on the carers, who reluctantly decided they could not continue with the placement.

I was asked to meet with the carers and the supervising social worker to see if the placement could be saved. Much of my thinking was about the challenges faced by young people of Vicky's age. Blos (1967) emphasised the push for autonomy, whilst Laufer and Laufer (1975) viewed the fundamental task for adolescence as the integration of the adult sexual body, believing that many of the difficulties faced by adolescents derived from this. Cregeen et al. (2017) refer to adolescence as a time for facing a rather abstract but intense kind of loss, the loss of childhood, sometimes experienced as the 'total loss of a psychic home'. This idea was particularly helpful in thinking about Vicky's experience.

Ironside (2009) reminds us that a young person's sense of self generally develops in the context of the birth family but in fostering it develops differently, i.e., within the context of loss, as well as with fresh opportunities for loving, being loved, healing and growth. Vicky's early years in care had provided many positive opportunities, which seemed to become lost in adolescence. As with most adolescents, the peer group took precedence. Horne (2009) writes that this group offers a variety of roles and opportunities to share responsibility and irresponsibility, trying out different aspects of the self and perceiving these in others. Unfortunately for Vicky, the peers came from similarly troubled backgrounds and drew her into activities that repeated the abuse and the neglect she had experienced as a child.

Wilson (1991: 186) refers to this tendency in adolescents to plunge into activities in order to find out and feel real but notes their difficulty in reflecting on experience and the limited capacity for self-observation. Bailey (2006) also notes that when carers become caught up in these adolescent difficulties, they can themselves become forced into action. The role of the therapist in such situations is not to advise on actions the carer should or should not take, rather to listen, make observations and connections, as this can be a source of support when carers feel powerless. In her 2017 study, Sloan Donachy writes about carers losing their sense of self and becoming disorganised and defensive. This was the case with Vicky's carers, who over time lost their previously held positive identity as successful and effective foster carers.

I met them without Vicky, and it was important that I began by acknowledging their anger, disappointment and disillusionment. This enabled the emergence of a reflective space in which they could begin to recall memories of the frightened, distressed eight-year-old they took in, who pined for her mother and needed much comfort and reassurance that she was not to blame for her situation. Over time, Vicky had begun to settle and make claims on them as parents, so her behaviour now was perceived as throwing their care back in their faces. As the session progressed, it was possible to talk about adolescents more generally and the psychological challenges they face in becoming separate from their parents, even though they are ill-equipped to manage the process. Klein (1957) saw adolescence as another chance to work over these fundamental issues of separation but, as Waddell (2000) points out, adolescence can also be a frightening time for young people and their carers, one in which creative developmental possibilities carry the fear of loss, including loss of the comparatively safe state of being a child.

The consultation, though helpful, did not save Vicky's placement, too much had happened, and she was moved to semi-independent accommodation. Nonetheless, it enabled the carers to remain in contact with her, which allowed some repair to take place between them, and ongoing contact with the organisation staff to be maintained. These links were important in preventing Vicky repeating her early experience of engagement with important objects, followed by abandonment. Her case was also helped by her eight years with carers who knew her story. With their ongoing support, albeit slightly distanced, the carers continued to provide a background of safety and to be attachment figures that Vicky could identify with as role models. The consultation to the team and the carers was a reminder that, for the child or young person in care, separation and individuation is never an easy process, as they have to mourn the loss of more than one set of parental figures on their journey to adult independence.

Vignette 2
Omar, 15, arrived in this country unaccompanied. He is from a Middle Eastern country and had lost contact with his parents. He was unsure if they were still alive. As a young person under 16, he came under the protection of social services and was placed with the organisation. In the initial team meeting much thought was given to the type of placement that would meet his needs. There was no cultural match for him, but the carer chosen had gained knowledge and relevant cultural understanding through looking after other asylum-seeking young people. Secondly, it was thought that, although from a different country, the presence of another asylum-seeking young person in the home could help to reduce the feelings of isolation that a lone young person might experience in placement. Burnett and Peel (2001) cite research about young Iraqi refugees in the UK that suggests depression is more closely linked with poor social support than with a history of torture. Omar was encouraged to link up with people from his own cultural group already in the UK, as this was seen as a useful way of sharing and making sense of his experiences. Making friendships and joining in activities with indigenous groups was also encouraged, as this can help build a sense of belonging to a new culture.

In placing young people such as Omar, there is an expectation that the organisation and carer will familiarise themselves with the structure and belief systems of the young person's country of origin. Similarly, it was important for me as consultant to have knowledge of different cultural models of mental distress and illness. As Helman (1994) reminds us, a person's response to a traumatic event can be shaped by their beliefs about self and identity and by cultural norms and attitudes to health and illness. Rack (1982) further warns against generalising too readily about refugees as a category, as there will be differences between them, depending on the country from which they come and their reasons for leaving. Whilst researchers such as Digidiki and Bhabha (2017) point to the remarkable resilience and coping skills seen in these young refugees, Melzak et al. (2018) explore their difficult experiences, both during and after arrival.

Much has been written about the symptoms often seen among the refugee popula-
tions – depression, anxiety, panic attacks – symptoms that come under the category
of post-traumatic stress disorders (PTSD). Omar has not been formally assessed for
PTSD, but he does have some related symptoms, i.e., nightmares, headaches and
problems with memory and concentration. Melzak *et al.* cite research that highlights difficulties in remembering and forgetting that can emerge after experiences
of traumatic violence and loss. An important part of my role as consultant was to
help the team to distinguish between behaviours that suggest serious mental ill
health from those that have a bearing on ordinary adolescent coping strategies.
Whilst Omar is prone to occasional angry outbursts and tends to overreact to minor
disappointments, this is partly due to his frustration at not being understood in
English and also may be a way of discharging pent-up feelings about his asylum
situation.

The focus in the organisation is on supporting Omar whilst he waits for the
Home Office decision on his application. Although these are early days in placement, the familiarity, consistency and containment provided by the carer are enabling a shift in his initial distrust of authority figures. Omar does not want to keep
going over the details of his experience en route to the UK, and my advice to the
team and the carer is not to challenge this, but to remain open, receptive and available to listen when opportunities for sharing arise. Melzak *et al.* draw attention
to some of the factors that help young people in Omar's situation to recover their
emotional equilibrium. Psychotherapeutic help is one, but this is not yet available
to Omar as a new arrival with uncertain asylum status.

Another factor that can work in a looked-after child's favour is the quality and
length of time during which they have experienced stable, secure relationships
within their birth family and community during the early years. There are signs
that Omar has had such experiences and is able to draw on them, which bodes well
for his recovery. A further factor in helping Omar to begin to process his trauma
is feeling safe and supported by the organisation. In terms of relevant adolescent
tasks, these may take longer to achieve and may in part rely on the successful resolution of his asylum claim. It may then be possible for sufficient mourning to take
place to enable Omar to confidently move forward in his development.

Conclusion

In this chapter, I have reflected on the role that a child psychotherapist can play
as a consultant in contexts surrounding children and young people in distress.
Throughout, the support of my peer supervision group has been invaluable in keeping me on task. The consultation is ongoing, and I have learned much in the process, as well as gaining a heightened appreciation for the team, foster carers and the
wider network who go the extra mile in addressing the needs of these very troubled
children and young people.

I would like to finish with a note on research. Blake and Moulton (1978) remind
us that consultation, in common with supervision, is not a scientific discipline; it
is largely fragmented, allowing various techniques to spring up, each carrying its

own tool kit. There is, currently, limited research-based evidence available on the effectiveness of consultation, the competencies and skills required. There has also been little examination of the nature and benefits of or barriers to collaborative consultation. For Gable et al. (2004), there is a dearth of guidance for practitioners, beyond what they have learned from responding to their clients' perceived need, or from interventions based on their own subjective bias. It is clear that research into the value and processes of consultation by a child psychotherapist could be a useful contribution to developing efficacy. However, I would argue from my own experience, and from the organisational outcomes, that the consultation process described in this chapter has enabled a change in practice among staff, which in turn has enhanced their practice with foster carers.

References

Akhtar S (1999) *Immigration and Identity: Turmoil, Treatment and Transformation* Northvale, NJ: Jason Aronson.
Bailey, T (2006) There is no such thing as an adolescent. In M Lanyado and A Horne (eds.) *A Question of Technique* London: Routledge.
Bion, W R (1962) *Learning from Experience* London: Karnac.
Blake, R R and Mouton, J S (1978) Toward a general theory of consultation. *Journal of Counseling & Development 56 (6)*: 328–330.
Blos, P (1967) The second separation individuation process of adolescence. *Psychoanalytic Study of the Child 22 (1)*: 162–186.
Burnett, A and Peel, M (2001) Health needs of asylum seekers and refugees. *British Medical Journal 322 (7285)*: 544–547.
Crawley, H (2007) When is a child not a child? *Asylum Age Disputes and the Process of Age Assessment* London: Immigration Law Practitioners Association.
Cregeen, S, Hughes, C, Midgley, N, Rhode, M and Rustin, M (2017) *Short-term Psychoanalytic Psychotherapy for Adolescents with Depression. A Treatment Manual.* J Catty (ed.) London: Karnac Books.
Digidiki, V and Bhabha, J (2017) *Emergency Within an Emergency. The Growing Epidemic of Sexual Exploitation and Abuse of Migrant Children in Greece* Harvard Kennedy School https:www.hks.harvard.edu/centres/cid/Publications
Douglas, H (2007) *Containment and Reciprocity: Integrating Psychoanalytical Theory and Child Development Research for Work with Children* Hove: Routledge.
Gabbard, G O (2000) Consultation from the consultant's perspective. *Psychoanalytic Dialogues 10 (2)*: 209–218.
Gable, S L, Reis, H T, Impett, E A and Asher, E R (2004) What do you do when things go right? The intrapersonal and interpersonal benefits of sharing positive events. *Journal of Personality and Social Psychology 87 (2)*: 228–245.
Gibbs, I (2006) A question of balance: working with the looked-after child and his network. In M Lanyado and A Horne (eds.) *A Question of Technique* London: Routledge.
Helman, C G (1994) *Culture, Health and Illness: An Introduction for Health Professionals,* Third edition, Oxford: Butterworth-Heinemann Reid Educational Professional Publishing.
Horne, A (2009) Normal emotional development. In M Lanyado and A Horne (eds.) *The Handbook of Child and Adolescent Psychotherapy: Psychoanalytic Approaches,* Second edition, London: Routledge.

Hunter-Smallbone, M (2009) Child psychotherapy for children looked after by local authorities. In M Lanyado and A Horne (eds.) *The Handbook of Child and Adolescent Psychotherapy: Psychoanalytic Approaches,* Second edition, London: Routledge.

Ironside, L (2009) Working with foster carers. In M Lanyado and A Horne (eds.) *The Handbook of Child and Adolescent Psychotherapy: Psychoanalytic Approaches,* Second edition, London: Routledge.

Kahn, W A (2001) Holding environments at work. *The Journal of Applied Behavioural Science 33 (3):* 260–279.

Kirby, J (2022) The difference between consultation and supervision. In *New Perspective Consultation & Supervision* https://newperspectiveconsultation.com/the-difference-betw een-consultation-and-supervision.

Klein, M (1957) *Envy and Gratitude* London: Virago.

Lanyado, M. (2009) The impact of listening on the listener: consultation to the helping professions who work with sexually abused young people. In A Horne and M Lanyado (eds.) *Through Assessment to Consultation* Hove: Routledge.

Lanyado, M (2017) Putting down roots: the significance of technical adaptations in the therapeutic process with fostered and looked after children. *Journal of Child Psychotherapy 43 (2):* 208–222.

Laufer, M and Laufer, E (1975) *Adolescent Disturbance and Breakdown* Harmondsworth: Penguin.

Melzak, S, McLoughlin, C and Watt, F (2018) Shifting ground: the child without family in a strange new community. *Journal of Child Psychotherapy 44 (3):* 326–347.

Ogden, T (2004) On holding and containing, being and dreaming. *The International Journal of Psychoanalysis 85 (6):* 1349–1364.

Rack, P H (1982) *Race, Culture and Mental Disorder* London and New York: Tavistock Publications.

Ruch, G (2011) Where have all the feelings gone? Developing reflective and relationship-based management in child-care social work. *British Journal of Social Work 42 (7):* 1315–1332.

Robinson F, Luyten, P and Midgley, N (2017) Child psychotherapy with looked after and adopted children: UK national survey of the profession. *Journal of Child Psychotherapy 43 (2):* 255–277.

Schein, E H (1990) A general philosophy of helping: process consultation. *Sloan Management Review 31 (3):* 57–64.

Sloan Donachy, G (2017) The caregiving relationship under stress: foster carers' experience of loss of the sense of self. *Journal of Child Psychotherapy 43 (2)* 223–423.

Sprince, J (2002) Developing containment. *Journal of Child Psychotherapy 28 (2):* 147–161.

Waddell, M (2000) Developmental issues from early to late life. *Psychoanalytic Psychotherapy 14 (3):* 239–252.

Wheal, A (1999) *The RHP Companion to Foster Care* London: Russell House Publishing.

Wilson, P (1991) Psychotherapy with adolescents. In J Holmes (ed.) *Textbook of Psychotherapy in Psychiatric Practice* London: Churchill Livingstone.

Winnicott, D W (1965) *Maturational Processes and the Facilitating Environment. Studies in the Theory of Emotional Development* London: Hogarth Press and Institute of Psychoanalysis.

Chapter 10

'A journey of a thousand miles begins with a single step …'

Teaching and supervising on a psychoanalytic training programme based in China

Coretta Ogbuagu

Like the baby who takes its first tentative step, a student of psychoanalysis can face a similarly daunting task, learning to balance moments of precariousness with an indomitable determination to rise to the challenge. This chapter will focus on the author's experience of this tension both in herself and for her students in an online weekly mother-infant observation seminar with a group of Chinese clinicians. Winnicott in his seminal paper 'Primitive emotional development' ([1945]1958) introduces three early developmental processes – (1) 'integration' (2) 'personalization' and (3) 'realization' – to describe the beginnings of our inner psychic reality. Using Winnicott's ideas, I will explore the dynamic process of student learning alongside observed infant emotional development, as well as discussing a parallel process within the seminar group. The inner workings of the seminar group and the outer reality of the Covid pandemic during this time made for a powerful teaching and learning experience.

The course

The Sino-British Programme is a three-year postgraduate training course for Chinese participants working as counsellors and psychotherapists with children and adolescents. It was developed and is delivered by Dr Viviane Green and Dr Qian Wang, who welcomed their first cohort in 2012. The course is focused on teaching and supervising qualified practitioners. It offers the opportunity for them to develop their practice and their understanding of psychoanalysis and apply it in a Chinese cultural context. I joined the teaching staff in 2018. I facilitate an online mother-infant observation (MIO) seminar group. Since 2018 there have been 16 MIO groups run by nine teachers. Each group begins with the commitment of a year, but most students will go on to observe for a further year until the child's second birthday. I have also been involved in delivering part of the teaching programme face to face in Beijing, including theoretical and clinical teaching and large group supervision. For the purposes of this chapter, I will focus on the supervisory aspect of my role as seminar leader to already qualified and established clinicians but who are new to the experience of parent-infant observation.

The MIO groups each consist of six students, plus an interpreter. The students join the group online from their individual homes or offices and they can be in

DOI: 10.4324/9781003297604-13

different states across China. One of my groups ran from July 2019 to July 2020 and so spanned the height of what started as a coronavirus epidemic in China and spread to become a pandemic across the globe. It was during this time that I visited Beijing to deliver teaching and supervision in person, though the observation seminars continued online as they always had. We now know that, as a group of teachers from the UK, we were there at the advent of the pandemic. Unfortunately, for my group of students, two group members were not successful in finding babies and the necessarily strict lockdown that took place in February 2020 in China just after their New Year celebrations did not help in this endeavour.

With the pandemic ongoing, my subsequent group began with minimal interference from a few local lockdowns in China. Thankfully, this did not prevent any group members from finding a baby to observe.

As a supervisor based in the UK, I face my own challenges running these online groups. Among them I observe the following:

- Technological challenges when the internet connection is unstable.
- Establishing a synchronicity with the interpreter – so that they come to understand my syntax and convey not only what I am saying but also the way in which I say it. I have noticed, for example, that I gesticulate often (such as demonstrating the holding of a baby), but the interpreter conveys my emphasis in words only, not by mirroring my gestures. Perhaps I find this more conspicuous because mirroring is what we hope parents will do with their young babies; matching facial expressions with the mood they feel the baby is expressing as a way of strengthening communication between them.
- Being aware of my assumptions about Chinese culture, including stereotypes and prejudices. It is interesting that in the UK Chinese and Black people are usually grouped together as a collective of ethnicities in the term BAME (Black, Asian and minority ethnic). Also in the UK, Chinese people are regarded as the 'model minority' (Chok 2018: 55; Loh 2018: 61 and Kam 2017: 89). I have to hold in mind the consideration that my students see me as a 'minority' and that they may have their own stereotypes about Black people – as well as, perhaps, some curiosity about me as a Black female teacher.

Cultural perspectives on learning

My own perception of the students falls in line with the 'model minority' stereotype: keen to absorb any knowledge and insights that can be shared in order to improve their ongoing clinical practice. I have the impression that they wish to be the best they can be. My own experience as a learner is that this takes time. One cannot grasp all there is to know about the psychodynamics of human interactions by the end of a course. In fact, I find that even now, many years on, I still reflect on my own infant observation experience and what I learned about the family I observed, how intense the experience was both in the family home and within the seminars with my peers and teachers.

I approach the task of supervision with the attitude of a learner. I expect to learn something from each encounter with the group. I expect to be surprised. I aim to be creative, and I challenge myself to think outside what might be considered the 'normal' way to do things, or the way they have always been done. Partly, this makes the experience livelier and more interesting for me, but also, this free-associative approach allows for spontaneity in the seminar, as one does not know how group members will respond.

By taking this approach, I have come to learn the following:

- Group work online in a different cultural setting from the one in which I am living brings challenges and is enlightening.
- Supervision is a process, and it requires trust. Trust takes time to develop.
- Supervising others is a craft and the peer-to-peer, as well as the student-teacher relationship, is central to the learning experience. In this I also include the teacher-to-teacher learning.
- Trying to learn about the emotional experience of new life through infant observation as a health pandemic is unfolding can be painful.

I would like to discuss the above points in more depth, drawing on Donald Winnicott's paper on 'Primitive emotional development' together with the Brazilian educator and philosopher Paulo Freire's ideas on power relationships in education as a reference point for understanding the dynamics at play in my work with the group.

It is worth having in mind some aspects of the Chinese context in which I supervise. Since opening up to foreign trade and investment and implementing free-market reforms in 1978, China has become known as one of the fastest growing economies in the world. Its evolution into a 'socialist market economy' means this generation of Chinese people are keen to learn and develop what they can from other so-called 'developed' nations around the world. In her 2021 article reflecting on the experience of setting up the teaching programme, Dr Green outlines the historical context in which we teach and its implications for the task of developing psychoanalytic ideas in China, as well as detailing the particular journey of cross-cultural teaching: teachers from the British schools of psychoanalysis and psychotherapy offering their knowledge to Chinese students. The mercantile attitude that Dr Green notes made its way into the MIO setting: students sharing that families were expecting payment for their time, or something tangible at the very least, such as a report or summary of their child's development.

In his theory of critical pedagogy, Freire argued that teaching should challenge learners to examine power structures and patterns of inequality embedded in society and culture, as well as in the processes of education. Education, he said, 'must begin with the solution of the teacher-student contradiction, by reconciling the poles of the contradiction so that both are simultaneously teachers and students' (Freire [1970]2017: 45). Freire's ideas derived from his experience of oppression in his early life and his observations of the teaching system (and its long-term impact) to which he and many others were and continued to be subject. Although I have an interest in his ideas, I note that his view is at odds with the Chinese Communist culture (despite its move towards capitalism), and the way the students of the Sino-British Programme are used to learning (Green 2021). Freire took issue with 'the banking system of education', which, he argued, consists of 'depositories' (students) and 'depositors' (teachers) ([1970]2017: 45). In this model of education, the teacher is the all-knowing font of wisdom and the students are empty containers which the teachers fill with what they know. Freire highlights the passivity in such an approach and how this serves to bring forth more of the same. 'The teacher cannot think for her students, nor can she impose her thought on them. Authentic thinking, thinking that is concerned about reality, does not take place in ivory tower isolation, but only in communication' (Freire [1970]2017: 50).

I agree with this idea and – apart from the adherence to what I think of as necessary structures of a teaching programme, such as group rules including respect for one another's views, punctual start and finish times and a format for how a seminar will be facilitated – I like to approach teaching from a creative, interactive perspective, encouraging an exchange of ideas and sharing of dilemmas, with space for both serious considerations and humour.

I have come to learn that what may be understood as 'funny' or 'humorous' in one culture, is not necessarily funny in another. Laughter can also serve as an expression of concealed anger or anxiety:

> A student made a comment and laughed. As I waited patiently for the student to finish and then the translation to follow, I noticed other members of the group laughed too, covering their mouths as if surprised. The translation was delivered and I realised that they were furious and empathised with the observer's predicament at feeling like a powerless witness to parenting they strongly disapproved of. One student asked if this was what the course was teaching: for them to observe difficult situations and say nothing to the family about this! 'Are we creating clinicians who are cold and cut off?'

Perhaps Winnicott can help us think here about the learning process for the student being mirrored by the developmental process for the baby.

Integration

Winnicott postulates a 'primary unintegration' for the infant at the very beginning of life and argues that 'the tendency to integrate' is dependent on his/her experience of ordinary infant care, together with instinctual experience. An infant needs to have all 'his bits and pieces' gathered together by someone (the primary caregiver, usually the mother) in order to begin to develop a sense of self and to be known. Without this, he/she cannot 'maintain integration with confidence' and may never succeed in this aim; causing issues in future relationships (Winnicott [1945]1958: 149–150).

A new learning experience brings a lot of uncertainty and huge expectations. At the beginning of the course, the MIO group ask the usual questions about how to find a baby to whom one is not closely connected, how to explain the task and the agreement for observing to the family and why anyone would agree to this. As time goes on and the group members find their babies, I need to hold on to their disappointed feelings: this is not the baby they hoped it would be, or the mother or father they hoped they would meet; the family are not very welcoming, or the baby is ignored, or 'Is this how my baby felt?' or 'How I felt as a baby?', or 'Is it how my parents felt about me?'.

Such feelings highlight the importance of the 'holding' function of the supervisor. The ability to manage the primitive anxieties and raw emotions that arise and can become magnified in a group setting. Sometimes students may join together as allies and form a union against the supervisor, who becomes the 'bad guy'. I understand this as an avoidance of processing difficult feelings. It becomes a useful defence mechanism to project the unwanted, unprocessed feelings on to the supervisor who represents the training institution. As a supervisor, it is my role to find a sensitive way of reframing what is projected on to me and sharing this with the group in a more digestible format. Doing this helps students to recognise the projections but does not aim to humiliate them in the process of coming to this awareness.

> A student presented their report and when I wondered about group reflections and comments, there was silence for a very long time. I waited a while, then wondered out loud what people were thinking. One brave student finally said that they came to hear what I had to say rather than share thoughts themselves. I was after all, 'the teacher'. I responded to what felt like a hostile accusation of me not doing my job properly by explaining how learning works in a group setting and how different ideas did not need to be fully formed or particularly clever or even 'right', nor did they all need to come from me. I proposed a way of working together which meant that the group could share their views with one another, then summarise this and share with me and then I could share my thoughts too. Perhaps a transactional approach? This allowed all voices to be heard and helped to avoid the aforementioned 'banking system' process that Freire referred to.

This is what I believe contributes to the trust that is co-created by students and supervisor over time. In the same way, a baby and its primary caregiver come to know one another through the repeated gathering together of the baby's fragmented experiences and expressions; these are then reflected back to him/her in a way that is less overwhelming and can be integrated into their sense of themselves and the world.

Personalization

Winnicott described 'satisfactory personalization', the feeling that 'one's person is in one's body' (Winnicott [1945]1958: 151), as building up over time through both instinctual experience and the 'quiet experiences of body-care'. The infant observation student will be witness to this process as they observe the baby each week (Sternberg 2005: 86). Being trained in the British Independent tradition of psychoanalytic psychotherapy, I come to the Sino-British Programme (and indeed all my work) with a view that, although I carry a psychoanalytic framework of reference in mind, I am still an individual and therefore unique. Some aspects of psychoanalytic thinking make sense to me, and others do not. How one perceives a baby in his/her environment will be coloured by one's own cultural understanding of child-rearing practices and rituals. I find as a supervisor in this situation I need constantly to re-evaluate my own Caribbean and British ideas about acceptable baby care, in an effort to be more useful alongside my Chinese students, as well as to learn from them about their practices and the reasons behind these, if known.

> While sharing an observation report, a student commented on how surprised they were to see that the family being observed followed the cultural rituals of hanging dog bones on the baby's pram. I asked what meaning this had. I was told that this is a traditional practice more likely to have been followed by previous generations and less so by the current one. The dog bones are said to ward off evil, protecting the baby.

As a Black British clinician, I bring a particular perspective to this supervisory relationship.

The programme itself has been developed by two women from different cultural backgrounds. A pedagogical community has been created because of these two forces joining together. Their openness to listening and making necessary adaptations has been much appreciated by teachers like myself. Their guidance and leadership have been crucial to the success of the programme. The American writer and critic bell hooks[1] emphasises the need for spaces for teachers to discuss and share their approaches to teaching in a cross-cultural context (hooks 1994: 37–38). I have found our teachers' meetings most useful as I came to learn that other teachers were facing similar challenges about experiential learning with students. I also noticed that the deference towards them from the students that many of the teachers described was largely alien to me. Perhaps this is because Chinese culture favours learning from elders – as demonstrated in the significant role grandparents take in agreeing the infant observations and making key decisions about the baby's care.

> When I met students in person in 2019, a group of them approached me whispering giddily amongst themselves. One summoned up the courage to ask how old I was and wondered at what age I began studying and training. How could I know so much but appear to be so young?

As a supervisor, as in other leadership roles, one receives many projections from others. I have found that being reminded of my apparent youthfulness could also be an unconscious communication about my ethnicity or race. Does it, in reality, represent the unspoken (and incredulous) question: 'How can you, as a Black person, know so much about this kind of work?' Similarly, I have wondered about another question often posed to me: 'How did you come to train as a child psychotherapist?' Why is it questionable for me to be interested in this work so early in life, yet acceptable for others, including great teachers and supervisors in this profession? Anna Freud herself began her psychoanalytic practice with children before she was 30 (Young-Bruehl 2008). Being grounded in one's sense of self – the personalization that Winnicott describes – seems as crucial to the development of the supervisor as it does to the emotional development of an infant. During online seminars, the lack of an embodied experience perhaps meant that students did not dare ask me certain questions directly. Conversely, students were sometimes very direct in their criticisms of the supervisor's approach. I wonder if they would have been so scathing if we were meeting face to face?

> During one seminar, I wondered if anyone had a view about the observation that had just been presented. After some silence, someone said with a wry smile, 'there is no democracy in China'. I took that to mean that, as the supervisor, I make the decisions and they will happily follow my lead. No collaborative teaching and learning here.

Realization

According to Winnicott, this important step in the early infantile process, beginning before the baby is six months old, is where reality meets fantasy. It concerns the infant's 'contact with external or shared reality' (Winnicott [1945]1958: 154). For example, if the infant is hungry and then expects milk, once the caregiver provides it, fantasy and reality meet. Winnicott posits that this meeting is a moment of healthy illusion because the baby has the experience of having created the breast/bottle, while at the same time 'his ideas are enriched by actual details of sight, feel, smell' of the experience (152). Over time, again as a result of consistent caregiving experiences, the infant is said to learn what is actually available in reality, thus becoming capable of making the distinction between fantasy and reality.

Like Winnicott's infant, the students arrive to both the observation setting and the group seminar with ideas about what they wish to create. It could be said that they bring their fantasies to our meetings. The learning comes when, as an observer, one realises that what is seen is different from what one thinks one has seen. This often comes to light in the group discussion when a variety of perspectives of the same situation are shared.

Sometimes, as mentioned earlier, the student may target criticism at the supervisor in response to being met with something they were not expecting. For Winnicott's infant, this would be the wish to attack and destroy the breast that delivers the milk, but then, once fed and gratified, a feeling of dissatisfaction persists because the plans for attack were not executed. Winnicott suggests that this could be why some infants are not happy at the end of a feed. I certainly recognise this feeling at the end of some seminars. Green (2021) writes about the importance, for the development of a psychoanalytic attitude, of staying with uncertainty, of fostering as a necessary clinical skill what poet John Keats termed 'negative cap-ability' (Gittings 1970: 43, letter of 21 December 1817) – an ability to tolerate not knowing later elaborated by various psychoanalysts, including Bion (1970: 125), Parsons (2000: 150) and Phillips (2010: 118–197). The coronavirus pandemic left us all facing the uncertainty of life in an unexpected way. My own experience of illusion meeting reality was, while back home in the UK, learning that the corona-virus was spreading across China but feeling initially that it was something distant. Try as I might, I could not believe the real-life stories I was hearing. Students explained why they could not observe face to face any longer and could not leave their homes except for a specific number of times a week to get food and so on. Then, Covid-19 arrived in the UK and everything I had been hearing in the last few months made much more sense. The anxiety expressed in different ways by the group in the previous two to three months was now much more within my field of understanding.

Sharing the uncertainty of life during this time brought us together in a unique way. I found myself drawing upon what seemed reasonable and flexible, rather than rigidly adhering to my usual frame of reference for teaching, supervising and learn-ing. 'Demonstrating critical social awareness and cultural humility allows super-visors and clinicians to build the trust and safety necessary to encourage growth across cultural and social differences', write Hernández and McDowell (2010: 29). The need for something personal, traditional and familiar became increasingly sig-nificant during this period. Anecdotal stories from my own circle of people about medicinal herbs and remedies to combat illness were reiterated as fail-safe ways of tackling any virus now or yet to come. I think I drew on this to understand that Chinese culture would likely have its own traditional views and ways of man-aging, and that following government instructions was one of these. Warren (2019) advocates the oral conveyance of information and experience in academia as a legitimate means of learning. We know that this is traditional practice in cultures across the world; stories are passed down orally from generation to generation and continue to have an impact. As far as the coronavirus pandemic is concerned, in one sense, the students and I had a shared reality.

I returned to my original thoughts about being used to being classified as 'other' in the UK, along with my Chinese counterparts. Surely, the students would also take solace in traditional, ancestral, tried and tested ways of managing uncertainty. It is hard to know how much of this derives from my own preoccupations and how much these feelings may have been shared with the students at the time. I will never know. I will never know how they observe me as a Black British teacher. Do they question if I know what I am doing? Do they believe they are getting a raw deal? Do they trust me? Am I a novelty to them?

At the end of a seminar group, I had been facilitating for a year, I asked the students for any feedback about their learning experience. After a long pause, someone said, 'I really liked your hair and the different styles and colours you wore.'

What has my hair got to do with infant observation or my supervisory style and skills? I was disappointed, but it helped me understand that there are prejudices in both directions and sometimes the observed 'object' being discussed is not necessarily the one we think.

Conclusion

Supervising a group of Chinese clinicians engaged in parent-infant observation has encouraged me to consider how Western theory and practice in psychoanalysis can be taught and applied to a different cultural context – in this case, modern-day China – and the challenges this may present. Furthermore, having what I would describe as a pluralistic and multifaceted identity (in its simplest form: Black, British and Caribbean) adds another layer of complexity to what happens in the psychodynamic relationship between the supervisor and those being supervised. Bringing together Winnicott's ideas on early emotional development, first published during the post-war period in Britain, and Brazilian Freire's ideas, published around the time of the so-called Chinese Cultural Revolution of the mid- to late 1960s, makes for an interesting blend of learning objectives. This lends itself well to the position an observer needs to take in their role: being aware of the layers of difference, the nuances, understandings, misunderstandings, mysteries and unknowns; being open to the powerful experience of all this swirling together in one's mind and body during the observation hour, then writing it up – putting into words the memories, flashbacks, smells, fears, excitements, hope, concern, joy, despair …

Freire talked about the power struggles that exist between the teacher and the student and advocated for a united struggle against oppression in education. This, he would argue is where true liberation is achieved. I am left with a similar feeling when I come to the end of a supervision group: what is most satisfying is not only that I may have imparted something useful, but that I in turn have gained from the experience – much like the mother of a child who is no longer a baby but grown, independent and able to walk wherever their feet may take them.

Note

1   This is the pen name of Black feminist author Gloria Jean Watkins, who deliberately kept it lower case in an effort to focus attention on the work rather than the writer

References

Bion, W (1970) Prelude to or substitute for achievement. In *Attention and Interpretation: A Scientific Approach to Insight in Psycho-Analysis and Groups* London: Tavistock.
Chok, V (2017) *Yellow*. In N Shukla (ed.) *The Good Immigrant* London: Unbound.
Freire, P (1970/2017) *Pedagogy of the Oppressed* London: Penguin Random House.
Gittings, R (ed.) (1970) *Letters of John Keats: A Selection* Oxford: Oxford University Press.

Green, V (2021) The Sino-British Programme: reflections on developing a psycho-therapy programme for Chinese participants working with children and adolescents. *Psychoanalysis and Psychotherapy in China 4 (2)*: 182–193.

Hernández, P and McDowell, T (2010) Intersectionality, power, and relational safety in context: key concepts in clinical supervision. *Training and Education in Professional Psychology 4 (1)*: 29–35

hooks, b (1994) *Teaching to Transgress: Education as the Practice of Freedom* London: Routledge.

Kam, W M (2017) Beyond 'good' immigrants. In N Shukla (ed.) *The Good Immigrant* London: Unbound.

Loh, D Y (2017) Kendo Nagasaki and me. In N Shukla (ed.) *The Good Immigrant* London: Unbound.

Parsons, M (2000) *The Dove that Returns, the Dove that Vanishes: Paradox and Creativity in Psychoanalysis* London: Routledge.

Phillips, A (2010) Negative capabilities. In *On Balance* London: Penguin.

Sternberg, J (2005) *Infant Observation at the Heart of Training* London: Karnac Books.

Warren, P W (2019) *Black Women's Narratives of NHS Work-Based Learning: An Ethnodrama* Oxford: Peter Lang.

Winnicott, D W ([1945]1958) Primitive emotional development. In *Collected Papers: Through Paediatrics to Psycho-Analysis* London: Tavistock.

Young-Bruehl, E (2008) *Anna Freud, A Biography*, Second edition, London: Yale University Press.

Chapter 11

Lost in transmission

Lydia Tischler

You may recall Humpty Dumpty's assertion to Alice (Carroll 1865) that words meant what he chose them to mean; the issue was simply whether he or words would be master. He ended with a resounding call to 'Impenetrability! That's what I say!'

In therapy – at least the talking kind – we often struggle with 'impenetrability', even when we not only speak the same language but when, for both of us (therapist and patient or trainee and supervisor) it is our mother tongue. What then is the additional complication when we teach in one language which is most often English, when our audience is not English and their knowledge of the language is variable? Or when English, the language in which we teach, is neither the teacher's nor the trainee's first language?

No doubt many readers are or have been teachers or trainees or perhaps both; and some have both taught and studied in a language other than their mother tongue. This also applies to me as my mother tongue is Czech but I trained in psychotherapy in England. My experiences of teaching abroad are all in countries formerly behind the Iron Curtain.

Here, I consider two interlinked aspects, language and the cultural setting in the widest sense as well as the culture of psychotherapy (in particular child and adolescent psychotherapy) – or more often the lack of a culture, reflecting a society's attitude to children, especially to their mental health.

Language

In the Czech Republic I had the advantage of being able to use my mother tongue. In Russia my knowledge of Czech helped, as the roots of the language are similar. I could understand a considerable amount when trainees presented their case material in Russian. The similarity of the languages, however, also has its dangers as in quite a few instances the same words have one meaning in Russian and another in Czech. In the Czech film *Kolya* (1996) a Russian boy ends up in the care of a grumpy Czech bachelor. In one scene during a public holiday when it was compulsory to hang out the Soviet red flag, Kolya is delighted to see a red flag on their house and keeps pointing to it with pleasure and pride: 'krasnaya vlajka!'

DOI: 10.4324/9781003297604-14

In Russian *krasny* or the feminine form *krasnaya* means red, while in Czech the word means beautiful. The man contradicts Kolya angrily and says that it is not a *krasnaya* (beautiful) *vlajka* (flag). For him it was anything but beautiful. I am not sure how this was translated in the subtitles, but I suspect the subtlety was lost in the translation. The scene expresses not only the total misunderstanding between the two but is a comment on the Russian occupation during which the film is set.

As far as language was concerned, communicating in the Czech Republic was not a problem; in Russia it was relatively easy; but in Estonia – the third country where I taught – it was altogether different. There was nothing familiar in the language whose roots are close to Finnish and Hungarian. Despite my facility in picking up languages – unfortunately getting lost with advancing age – during my regular visits to Estonia over a period of two years I unusually never did learn even a smattering of the language.

Teaching psychoanalytic psychotherapy involves learning about another language, the language of the unconscious. This is a very special kind of learning which is difficult even in one's mother tongue, let alone when teacher and trainees don't speak the same language. It is difficult because it is to do with feelings or, more precisely, with emotions for which words are the vehicles, representing as they do drives and their derivatives and, as Freud taught us, they succumb to childhood amnesia. It is the language of our first relationships, the language we learnt from our mothers, and because it is the language of early childhood, it is also permeated with infantile fears and phantasies and knowledge which we thought we were not allowed to have. It is permeated with the inevitable anxieties belonging to psychosexual development.

Additionally, teaching psychotherapy creates a particular complex organisational dynamic between the trainers and those being trained. It is a paradox that the aim of psychoanalytic psychotherapy is to free the individual from unresolved unconscious and infantile conflicts and thus allow greater inner freedom, while the very process of training tends to infantilise its candidates and creates a culture of dependency. This can be even more accentuated when the teachers are 'foreigners' and the know-how has to be imported from abroad. Not only that, but often their services are given gratis or for a much-reduced fee. Both envy and gratitude come into play here.

The Lost Childhood and the Language of Exile (Szekacs-Weisz and Ward 2004) is an expanded version of papers given at a conference organised by Judith Szekacs, the founder of East-West Imago. Before the fall of the Iron Curtain, East-West Imago was a venue where therapists and analysts could come and talk about the often clandestine analytic activities that were going on in their countries. It was in fact through one of those chance encounters at a lecture given by the Czech analyst Michael Šebek that I was invited to set up a training in child and adolescent psychotherapy in Prague.

I have often pondered my motives for being so keen to teach in the Czech Republic, apart from the fact that, as I speak Czech, I spoke the same language as the course participants. While preparing this paper, I revisited Szekacs and Ward and, dealing as they do with lost childhood, it struck me that one of my underlying motives was looking for *my* lost childhood. Perhaps this is why so many expatriates have felt the urge to teach in their former home countries – seeking something we have lost. However, the conscious purpose was to bring psychoanalytic thinking and practice to countries who had lost it or where it was suppressed because it did not suit the prevailing regime, as in the Czech Republic where psychoanalysis flourished before the Second World War, and in Russia where it had also taken root before the revolution. Estonia, as far as I know, did not have an analytic tradition and there the wish to import psychoanalytic thinking came via a different route – again, through an expatriate:

> In 1995 Nils Taube invited John Schemilt, Gillian Dean and George Crawford to visit Estonia. Mr. Taube, an Estonian by birth, was involved with other western business people in supporting the rebuilding of the Estonian economy following the country's declaration of independence in 1991. He invited us to explore the possibility of helping to develop therapeutic services for children in Estonia along the lines of the work we were doing at the Scottish Institute of Human Relations.
> (Crawford 2004)

Supervision in another tongue

Having one's analysis in another tongue (*vide* Hoffman 2004) carries issues for our trainees that, as teachers, we must keep in mind. There is a crucial difference, however, with supervision since in analysis there is a dyad and in supervision there is a third but absent participant – the patient.

In supervision we inevitably get a second-hand account: the *actual* session cannot be recreated. The success of conveying the session will depend on the capacity of the supervisee to transmit accurately what went on in the session and on the supervisor's receptiveness. Supervision has long been a subject of study, especially issues of transference and counter-transference. It becomes much more complicated when therapist and patient speak one language (the therapy is conducted in their own language) and the therapist has then to report it in another language – in this case English. As English is also not *my* mother tongue but is my everyday language, I am perhaps more attuned to the struggles of conveying something for which supervisees do not have enough words or perhaps not the right words. Of course, the affective tone is of help in disentangling what is going on in the therapy room; however, the limitation of the language does create additional problems. This was especially the case in Estonia where I became aware how much of the subtlety of the interaction was lost not only in translation but in transmission in conveying the session.

In Estonian the grammatical construction is also very different from English and this adds to the difficulties:

> He wants to start pelt, but I stopped him, and said, that do not let, and did ask, why he wants to do so?

-Then father does afraid?
What father does afraid then?
I do afraid!
We go towards the door and he strikes me from the hair wery strongly, saying I do you Mi- tuti- (what is for very-very tender pulling).
-You not want to go away, but our time is ower, we can not help!

And from a report entitled 'At the bottom of the words':

Lisa start to walk towards someone else room and 'Mother does catch her and begins to dress off her', Mother is asked to wait in the hall. In the room 'there is a yellow plume on the table and I do blow on that'. The plume does flow by the table and Lisa likes this scene very much. She tries to blow herself but she can't then tell me to blow again. So we have a game I blow she is glad. It appears that mother can't stand Lisa enjoying herself with someone else this is what the therapists says next. Mother in the hall can't wait more, comes to the door, and does ask to enjoy.

(Rander 2005)

The supervisee has a double task, first of all to convert and then to convey. I had a discussion on just this topic with one of my former supervisees from Estonia, when she was on a short visit to England. I was curious to know what the experience of having to have supervision with me in English had been like and I got an unexpected answer. She said that not knowing English well enough made her feel stupid but she did not mind because she had to relate material in a foreign language; had she been bringing her material in Estonian to an Estonian supervisor, she would have minded not knowing. After supervision with me, she could translate our session into her own language and so had two chances to process and understand the patient's material, suggesting that this was something positive. Now, on reflection, I think we were not talking about the same thing: she was more concerned with what she felt were her inadequacies as a therapist, while I was interested in the limitations I presumed she felt in having to present the material in English. It seems that something got lost in transmission. However not all things get lost, sometimes they are also found. The same supervisee, Reet Montonen (who sadly died after a relatively short struggle with cancer), amongst her many important contributions to the development of child psychotherapy in Estonia, gave a report to a European Federation for Psychoanalytic Psychotherapy (EFPP) conference held in Tallinn in January 2005.

I quote two excerpts here:

I would like to start with a little vignette. It concerns a topic such as **weather.** Pilt talvest [a picture of winter].

    On one hand it is a very common topic – if you have nothing else to talk about or if you have too much to talk about then weather is a good subject. Still, the actual weather has influenced our training pretty much – we have had to cancel our meetings or changed them, it has been a subject in our seminars, caused quick visits to shop, etc. A long, cold, frosty and icy (slippery) winter has been especially influential. Especially for teachers. [I think Reet was referring to flights that were cancelled or delayed because of bad weather or because the one and only aircraft developed a fault. I recall one occasion when we arrived at 3am instead of 11pm – LT.] But a warm and friendly summer has always followed.

On the other hand, climate as creating an atmosphere needed for the new ideas to root. Weather and climate does not mean only the things we see and feel, but also the local and by that I mean Estonian possibilities, needs, resources etc. Creating a favourable climate for the project to succeed. As a conclusion we might say that the difficulties we faced in the beginning of the long training melted into pleasant cooperation and development.

(Montonen 2005)

She continues:

Just as important as the weather is another aspect – **the language.** The whole studying process was in English. It is a foreign language for all of us and our level of English is very different – we know different amount **words.**

Language is not only about words but also concepts, metaphors and ideas. It is very hard to communicate and express your ideas if you don't have the means. That rises anxiety and tension. The students and the teachers both know how important a subtle train of thought or use of words may be and how sad it is when it's not understood. A picture comes to my mind immediately – our teachers sitting and listening to us with their 'third ear'. All the senses are used to understand. And we keep explaining and explaining using various approaches to make a word or expression clear. Suddenly we realise that by explaining we have started to discuss and interpret the cultural-historical-political, etc., context.

(Montonen 2005)

The cultural environment

Differing cultural assumptions have led often to misunderstandings, sometimes sorted out, sometimes not. Supportive professional structures taken for granted in Scotland have been frequently lacking in Estonia and their absence has created many frustrations and difficulties for our trainees in establishing settings suitable for psychotherapeutic work. Perhaps more familiar to tutors coming from Great Britain has been a wider professional apathy towards and misunderstanding of psychoanalytical approaches to work with children.

(Crawford 2004)

In many countries in Eastern Europe, therapeutic work with children is not a high priority. It seems that, historically, emotional disturbance in children tends to go

> unrecognized or, when recognized, is likely to be treated pharmacologically. …
> Lack of awareness of the emotional needs of children of course leads to lack
> of interest in and funding for training in psychotherapeutic work with children.
>   (Report of the EFPP Child Section meeting, Prague Conference 2001)

The setting up of a training programme in Estonia had been a long, drawn-out process. Introductory talks had been attended by approximately 100 participants and we ended up with a group of eight candidates who qualified in 2004.

The process was somewhat different in the Czech Republic, where adult analysis and psychotherapy had been re-established quickly after the Velvet Revolution of 1989. Psychoanalysis had flourished before the Second World War, founded by Russian émigré analysts. It continued underground during the communist regime and, after the Velvet Revolution, it could once again exist in the open. I was invited to help set up a child and adolescent training programme for which the expertise was lacking in the Czech Republic.

My first encounter was in November 1994 when I met a group of interested child psychiatrists and psychologists to consider the feasibility of setting up a training programme. Judging by their response, my expectations were to say the least very different from theirs. In my enthusiasm and somewhat omnipotently I had in my mind the establishment of a training programme that would be based on the Association of Child Psychotherapists (ACP)'s 'Outline for trainings'. This document sets out the requirements which established training schools are expected to follow and new trainings must put in place. These included personal therapy four times a week for the duration of the training, weekly observation of an infant for two years, three intensive training cases (an under-five, a latency child and an adolescent) seen three times a week, one for two years and two for one year, each supervised weekly by a different supervisor. We immediately stumbled on a problem. I was told very politely but in no uncertain terms that there was no way these requirements could be met. Infant Observation, a core part of the training in the West, was out of the question for a number of reasons. For a country so recently liberated from a 'Big Brother' regime, the idea of a stranger coming to observe mother and infant in the home would raise far too many paranoid anxieties; additionally access to families for observation could only be gained via the paediatricians and this also did not seem feasible. Most cases were seen once a week, at most twice weekly and only rarely seen for two years. Some quick thinking was necessary if we were not to falter at the first hurdle. Should I insist on the whole package or do I compromise and work with what is possible?

In my training as a psychotherapist I learned to meet the patient on the level at which he is able to engage with me. I believe it is a useful axiom, and that it applies equally to social situations when to ignore local conditions and customs will at best stifle any progress and at worst will be an imposition of one's own pre-conceived ideas, a form of mental colonisation. This axiom is a good corrective to one's omnipotence and missionary zeal. On that occasion, reality prevailed and a dialogue began which, after much work on both sides, turned wishful thinking into a practical reality. Our first visit to Prague took place in February 1996.

Potential course members were psychoanalysts or candidates of the Psychoanalytic Institute of the Czech Study Group of the European Psychoanalytical Federation of Psychotherapists, with the great advantage that all of them were in personal psychotherapy and already had a grounding in psychoanalytic theory and con-cepts. The Czech training therefore had a head start. It also had the advantage that I spoke Czech and that made it possible for members of the group whose English was not fluent enough to have supervision of their cases in their native language. However, this also created its own problems and tensions in the group between those who had a good command of English and understandably felt resentful that they were being slowed down by the necessity to translate the lectures – which were all delivered in English – for those who could not follow English. In this respect, the process was the reverse of the Estonian experience where it started with a wider public from which a core group remained. One other difference needs to be noted. The Estonian training was funded by Nils Taube but no such benefac-tors were available for the Czech training, though we did have funding from the British Council for the first two meetings, and subsequently our fares and accom-modation were paid from the course fees and the course leaders received some pocket money.

Although we had the blessing of our professional organisation, the ACP, it was not in a position to offer any more tangible support. The fact that we were not linked to and did not represent any of the training schools had both advantages and disadvantages. The disadvantage was not being able to call on an organisation's resources and support for us as trainers as no organisation could take this fledging training under its wing nor, importantly, provide it with the status of being linked to an established training programme as was the case with the Estonian train-ing which was linked to the Scottish Institute; to some extent this also applied to the training in St Petersburg where a basic training programme was provided by a group of therapists from the Anna Freud Centre. On the plus side, not being linked to a training school gave us the freedom to invite guest speakers from a wider spectrum of theoretical orientations. Over the years speakers came from the Anna Freud Centre, the British Association of Psychotherapists and the Tavistock Clinic.

Working conditions

The setting

While the newly founded child training programme had a place within the Czech Society for Psychoanalytic Psychotherapy (CSPP) structure, it lacked an infrastructure and a physical base such as a clinic or clinical service with its own referral network which could provide suitable training cases for its candidates; a multidisciplinary team that could offer assessment and provide work with parents; and a suitably equipped therapy rooms for children.

External factors

The group consisted of more or less experienced independent practitioners with variable skills in their core professions, working in diverse mental health settings, often in unfavourable external conditions within a medical hierarchy and in a treatment culture which, if not inimical, often did not place any value on a psychoanalytic perspective. Similar situations can obtain – though fortunately less frequently – for our trainees in the UK. However, there the training schools can offer more support and protection to the trainees in their clinical placements.

The work setting very often did not provide a suitable room to establish a therapeutic space with appropriate boundaries and suitable play material. Both in Prague and Estonia – and this applies to most countries from the former Soviet blocs who are struggling to establish training – rooms often have to be shared with other professionals and are often unsuitable for conducting psychotherapy. I recall one trainee in Estonia having to work in a hospital which was also a drug dependency unit and where the children had to step over discarded needles to get to their appointments.

Psychological factors

Learning involves integration of new knowledge: learning about psychoanalysis not as an academic subject but as a personal experience involves giving up defences; confronting ghosts from the past; letting go of outdated ideals and idealised objects; facing loss; feeling vulnerable, and for professionals there is the additional narcissistic injury of feeling temporarily deskilled. It involves giving up certainty, however restricting and stifling, and tolerating not knowing. In short it is a process involving psychic pain. It is a difficult process at the best of times; it is much harder when simultaneously familiar external structures are being dismantled. In the Czech Republic the political changes, which began with Perestroika in Russia and culminated in the Velvet Revolution, had a profound effect on the identity in its many layers and facets both of the individual and of society. The problems of identity have been of especial interest to psychoanalysts in the Czech Republic who had personal experience of growing up in a totalitarian regime even while they were resisting its influence. They have written extensively and cover such aspects as the ramifications on family life, intergenerational conflicts and the upbringing of children. It is a fascinating and complex issue and was the subject of the Czech Society for Psychoanalytic Psychotherapy Conference in Prague in May 1998 entitled 'Identity in post-totalitarian reality'. The conference proceedings were published in the Czech journal *Revue* in 1999. The impact of the totalitarian regime could also be felt in the seminars where there was an absence of a critical attitude to what was taught, and it took some time before participants felt free to think and question our assumptions.

Clearly different countries have dealt differently with the impact of a repressive regime. Sandra Linford writes of her Lithuanian experience:

> I remain troubled by their attitude to history and by their working with people while incorporating neither their own nor their patients' history into their work. Our cultural difference resides perhaps in the value we give to history in contrast to the way in which history has been anaesthetised in Lithuania.
>
> (Linford 2003)

Establishing a therapeutic relationship

The role of supervision

We considered supervision to be the most important contribution we made to the training and the participants themselves also valued this most highly. This was equally true in St Petersburg where I was able to travel from Tallinn for a day's supervision. However, these were not formal training supervisions where cases are carefully selected and approved as suitable by the supervisor. They were part of the individual caseloads and varied in severity of pathology and family sophistication.

Those of us who trained in England take it for granted that children have their own inner world which we as therapists respect, and we know their experiences of external reality will have been to a lesser or greater degree influenced by their inner drives and psychic reality, and their internalised relationships to their objects. Not only do we take for granted that they have their own internal world but also that they are entitled to it and in therapy we engage with it. Of course, children are not free agents and they come into therapy because someone – usually parents or teachers – is concerned for them. It is usually the external environment that suffers. When we began meeting with supervisees, the therapists saw themselves more as educators and agents of the parents, taking on the parents' agenda to 'make the problem go away'. The idea that the therapist could be a transference object for the child was at first difficult to accept, as was the idea that the child had his own perception of the world which needed to be understood, and that they had to deal not only with the real parent but also with the internalised parent of the child. This was reflected in their dealings with the parents and the physical setting provided for the patient. Inviting parents into treatment rooms did not seem out of the ordinary and the room itself was often unsuitably furnished with other patients' drawings displayed on the wall. Taking phone calls during a child's session was not unheard of.

Conclusion

The participants should, I think, have the last word. This is how Ivana Ruzickova, one of the Czech course co-coordinators, summarised the changes that have taken place:

> Gradually we are finding a new approach to theoretical thinking and a psycho-dynamic way of working is developing. A substantial shift is occurring as we learn to really see the child as our client and the centre of our attention. The changes that have taken place are very noticeable.
>
> (Ruzickova 2001)

Reflecting on the three years that had elapsed between two EFPP conferences, the first on the theme of 'Therapeutic space and containment', the second on 'Internal objects and psychic change', she conjectures that:

> during this time a similar process of availability of therapeutic space to the internalisation of the object took place in a group of likeminded professionals.
>
> (Ruzickova 2001)

And:

> From my personal experience I can vouch for the significance of having supervision. I cannot stress enough the special significance that the supervisions with Lydia Tischler and Miranda Feuchtwang had, during which the reality of transference and countertransference emerged. I learnt to listen to own my feelings, not to underestimate their importance but to work with them in therapy.
>
> (Ruzickova 2001)

And, finally, the voice of Reet Montonen:

> An important context should be included here – **the psychoanalytic thinking** that was new for us. All the words, notions and we needed to be connected to it. Common language in its widest sense was the key factor to make the studying process successful. One possibility in this field was the so-called Estonian English, which was acquired pretty well by our teachers also. A lot of our studies have been connected to **the emotional experiences.** New techniques, new theories, new ways of thinking. It often rises a question for us – what does it mean for me as a specialist, where should I put it, what am I going to do with it? How did it change us? How did it change our work?
>
> With confidence we can say – we changed and our work has been changed. During this development we became capable of spending 45 minutes with a

child and thinking together with the child. The truth is that child psychotherapy is an emotional work, is a very active work. Transferring relationship is basic – **to bear, to carry, to share.**

Freedom to think and to feel. The children have to be inside us, for us to be able to understand them.

Like George Crawford often said: 'We have to give the child a chance to be experienced, understood, seen etc. the way he/she is – in good and in bad.' This is a whole new level to be with the child. And it is important not to get tired, get frightened or give up. To bear the transference.

(Montonen 2005)

I have given Reet the last word as she so eloquently expressed the difficulties as well as the gains of becoming a child psychotherapist and how the problems of language and culture could be overcome. It is the internalisation of a psychoanalytic stance, a spirit of enquiry and curiosity, which her Czech and Russian counterparts also stressed as the important and lasting achievements. One cannot ask for more.

Note

This chapter is based on a talk given at the Multi-Lingual Psychotherapy Centre (MLPC) on 9 February 2008.

References

Carroll, L (1865) *Alice's Adventures in Wonderland* London: Macmillan.

Crawford, G (2004) Ventures and adventures in Estonia. In *Scottish Institute of Human Relations Newsletter 15.*

Grinberg, L (1997) Transference and counter-transference and the technique of supervision. In B V Martindale, M Morner, M E Rodriguez and J-P Vidit (eds.) *Supervision and Its Vicissitudes* London: Karnac.

Hoffman, E (2004) Lost and found in translation. In J Szekacs-Weisz and I Ward (eds.) *The Lost Childhood and the Language of Exile* London: Imago East-West and The Freud Museum.

Linford, S (2003) Teaching in Lithuania – the personal and the professional: the role of the counter-transference, unpublished paper.

Montonen, R (2005) *Child psychotherapy in Estonia – past and present.* Paper presented at the 3rd EFPP Conference for Central and Eastern European Networks, Tallinn.

Rander, M (2005) *At the bottom of the words.* Paper presented at the 3rd EFPP Conference for Central and Eastern European Networks, Tallinn.

Ruzickova, I (2001) *Child and adolescent training in the Czech Republic.* Paper presented at EFPP Conference of Central and Eastern European Networks, Prague.

Szekacs-Weisz, J and Ward, I (2004) *The Lost Childhood and The Language of Exile* London: Imago East-West and The Freud Museum.

Tischler, L (2001) *The problems of training: a view from the West.* Paper presented at Federation for Psychoanalytic Psychotherapy Conference of Central and Eastern European Networks, Prague.

Chapter 12

Mirrors to ourselves

Reflections on peer group supervision

Deirdre Dowling

Individual and peer group supervision are the backbone of continuing professional development, the ongoing support for many child psychotherapists after qualification. Peer groups also provide a peer monitoring system within the profession. Many of us stay with the same group for years and turn to the people there at moments of difficulty or stress in our career. The Covid pandemic sent these in-person groups online, which changed the dynamic, perhaps permanently. Online meetings created ease of access for those living at some distance from the group's former home and allowed us to meet at a critical time when we needed each other's support, but I find these online meetings have lost some of their vitality and intimacy, and I miss the personal contact.

The challenge and pleasure of psychotherapy is that each troubled young person we meet brings new clinical dilemmas, possibly ones we have not met before. However experienced we are, we can find ourselves at a loss, unsure how to understand the underlying causes of a child's distress or how to get through to help them when faced by their distrust or despair. Perhaps this is the reason that belonging to a peer group for supervision, alongside individual consultation, has always been such an important support in my work.

In this chapter, I would like to explore the value and potential pitfalls of this important forum for supervision. I could find little written about its contribution to our development as child psychoanalytic psychotherapists, so I have based this chapter on my own experience, but it would be interesting to know about the lives of the myriad other groups, and how they differ from my recollections. The peer group I attend have added their ideas to my original version, which I have woven into the discussion.

An introduction to peer group supervision

The majority of the writers in this book explore the value of the individual supervisory relationship. While I find this essential, peer group supervision offers something different. Essentially it is a leaderless group with the shared task and goal of offering a reflective space where members, in turn, can bring their cases for discussion and exploration. I am a long-term member of a child psychoanalytic group

DOI: 10.4324/9781003297604-15

with others from a variety of training backgrounds but with a shared analytic view-point. More recently, I also helped set up a local, mixed, interprofessional group of colleagues working therapeutically with children, who support each other with their work, bringing their different perspectives. Each of these groups offers some-thing different, but in this chapter, I will concentrate on the former, though much of what I will say is relevant to both.

Form and structure

An image that comes to mind to illustrate how the peer group functions when it works well is that of a community garden; a collaborative venture by a group or community who all want it to flourish, who feel a shared responsibility for its future and who each make a different contribution. One member is an expert on plant species, another on design, there are diggers and weeders and those who like to sit and admire it. Similarly in a group, we all bring different perspectives and skills that contribute to the shared task. The pleasure of a joint venture, doing this work together, is a bonus, but it is the common focus that creates the group alliance.

As a therapist, I have always enjoyed working in a group setting, observing how the group is able to develop a way of understanding that is deeper than each individual and to offer this as support. I am fascinated by the way that unconscious communi-cation between individuals facilitates ideas developing and allows complex feelings to be explored, at one step removed from the participants in the shared group space.

The support of a peer group can act as a balance to the solitary work of indi-vidual psychotherapy. For those working privately, it provides a team not of work colleagues but of fellow practitioners, who share the uncertainties and continual challenge of this work. However, for a leaderless group to be successful, there must be common assent to an agreed form and structure to provide reliability and safety. In my experience, a small group numbering 6–8 people works well. The meeting, often fortnightly or monthly, can last for 75–90 minutes, and is held at a regular time and place. In our group, we plan ahead who is to present a case each month, rather than leave the time open for requests on the day, as happens in some groups. Our approach allows time for the discussant to prepare detailed notes, which we find enables a depth of analysis not possible otherwise.

If these boundaries are not kept to, and individuals regularly turn up late or miss several sessions without notice, there is usually a protest, as the group no longer feels so reliable or safe. Typically, this will be taken up by members of the group and our agreement is confirmed again. In a newer group, it may take time to estab-lish these norms, but once a group culture develops, a pattern is established that helps ensure its continuity.

When we met in person, the meeting usually began with a brief drink and a snack when we arrived at our regular meeting place. The hostess played an important role in making us comfortable, preparing food and giving us a room to meet in after a long day at work. Then, as now, we would check in with each other how everyone was doing before we focused on the task in hand. It is a relief to share news and relax, and this creates the informal atmosphere that allows the group to be open with each other in the discussion that follows.

An agreed format is followed in each meeting, similar to that of individual supervision. Typically, the presenter outlines the family history of a child and an account of a clinical session uninterrupted, usually citing the problem they need help with. Sometimes the initial background and history is left until after the discussion of the clinical session. This allows the group's imagination to range among many possibilities that might be limited by knowledge of the chronology. Either way, the presenter then sits back and allows others to think about the material. If presenters intrude too much, then their perspective takes over, and new ideas cannot so easily arise. There may be questions at first, for clarification, and a discussion of the family history; then these thoughts are put aside while we listen to the session. Ideas begin to flow as one person's ideas sparks thoughts in another. These weave together until some resolution is reached towards the end, and the therapist is given ideas to take home for future work.

'A culture of enquiry'

This phrase was used by Tom Main (1983) to describe an essential quality of therapeutic community living, in which every aspect is open to question by the members, in order to explore and understand the complex relationship between our inner and outer life, as individuals and as a group. I think it can also be used to describe the free-ranging exploration and discussion of a clinical case in group supervision, moving between the patient's inner and outer worlds, the therapist's countertransference and the dynamic of the therapeutic relationship, inner conflicts and social and cultural realities. The range of life and work experience brought by each member of the group to the exploration of a complex case can reveal many threads that may not discovered in a two-person supervision. Each person will have their own counter-transference response to the child and family, giving added depth and breadth to the discussion. It is always fascinating to track the conversation as our thinking bounces off one another and themes emerge which can coalesce to a different way of understanding. I will share an example to illustrate this process. I have given limited details and altered facts to disguise the patient and maintain confidentiality. My focus is on the group process.

A clinical example

I recall presenting my difficulties with a new patient, I will call Charlie, aged 14. He had recently arrived in England from Australia, so he was new to the school system in England. He was on medication for anxiety and attention deficit hyperactivity disorder (ADHD) and he had been in intensive psychotherapy in his own country. There was a query as to whether he was on the autistic spectrum. When he was referred for therapeutic help, he was already in trouble for being disruptive in class and had been sent home on a warning. In the early psychotherapy sessions,

Charlie was angry and dismissive of my help, either responding with one-word answers or with prolonged silence. I felt intimidated, and at a loss as to how to make a connection with him. This was particularly hard as we had begun our work online due to the pandemic, so I missed the many nonverbal clues and the feeling for our relationship I would have picked up if we had met in person. Online, Charlie sat back on the sofa in his bedroom ignoring my questions and attempts to make conversation. He appeared distracted, probably playing on his mobile phone.

In the supervision group, I gave a brief history and described a session full of non sequiturs, feeling rather embarrassed by my inability to engage him in a conversation. Once my presentation was complete, there was silence at first and I felt more awkward, as if the group did not know how to respond to my uncertainty. Then members of the group took up different threads. One asked more about the worried parents, and their history, another commented on Charlie's loss of his home, his culture and friends. We discussed his psychiatric history and how he was seen by his previous therapeutic team. Finally, one long-term member of the group, who had known me for years, asked why I was so anxious and perplexed. She pointed out that I had dealt with many young people like him over the years and wondered how he could have got under my skin.

This led to more discussion about my counter-transference, and how I had absorbed Charlie's panic, anger and shame at his predicament. He feared exploring his feelings as he so easily felt overwhelmed. The group began to focus on his autistic defences against these complex feelings, complicated by the loss of his home, friends and culture. Like him, I had felt alone, and scared that we would not be able to build a therapeutic alliance. Then I would not be to help him begin to think about his difficulties and contain his anxieties in time to stop him having another meltdown at school and possible expulsion.

Exploring these issues with others helped contain my anxiety. I recognised the pressure on myself to succeed quickly, to rescue the young man. This was from his parents, for whom I felt great sympathy, and from the school, as well as Charlie himself. By giving me some emotional distance, the group discussion allowed me to begin thinking again. I realised I needed to get separate support for his parents and seek an alliance with the school, as he would need their patience and understanding through this early difficult phase. This would help me feel less isolated, as I would become part of a team around the child, and this could mirror my experience of feeling held in the group by our shared thinking.

Thoughts about the group process

The reflective process

I have noticed that the reflective process we see in individual supervision can occur in groups., where the dynamics of the case become mirrored in the supervisory pair. Temporarily, the members may be struck silent, as I think they were briefly in my session, hearing my anxiety and the child's panic. Similarly, the despair of a suicidal teenager or the uncomfortable resonances of a perverse interaction may be deeply felt by the group and take some time to process. Once someone is able to recognise and draw attention to this effect, the group is freed up to analyse their response and try to understand what is being communicated. An atmosphere of trust is needed for such honesty about one's feelings and to question another's response. But if this is possible, the group can become a creative space in which it is possible to try out new ideas or challenge accepted ones. Mani Vastardis and Gail Phillips describe eloquently how, in their supervision sessions, such case discussion may go in many different directions before coming to some conclusions.

> [We] struggle with our thoughts which are not necessarily beautiful and orderly, but can be resolutely untamed: interrupting, defying, refuting, contradicting not only the other person's thoughts, but even our own, in other words moving between two planes of thought in a wildly dionysiac dance.
>
> (Vastardis and Phillips 2012: 105–106)

Importance of the leaderless group

Early in the history of my participation in the group, when several of us were newly qualified, we decided to invite respected teachers to a series of sessions, so that we could develop our skills. Although it was exciting to have a well-known child psychotherapist in our midst, facilitating the discussion and bringing ideas, we eventually discontinued this. I can still remember how much I learnt from each of these teachers, but we also rather regretfully realised that the group had lost something in the process of having a facilitator and we returned to relying on our own skills. Looking back, I wonder if we knew that we would not develop confidence in our own growing capacity in supervision if we sat back and looked for expertise elsewhere. Also, I think we discovered that it is the wide-ranging thinking of a diverse group trying to problem-solve together that we enjoyed, rather than a particular viewpoint, however good.

Without a leader, the group has to deal with problems as they arise, as they are bound to over time, and achieve a consensus if we face disagreements. Issues such as inviting new members or changing the format of the sessions can create dissension. Once or twice in our group, we have used a vote to decide an issue when we could not come to a clear agreement, but this did not feel very satisfactory as it meant we had been unable to resolve our differences. The group also has to be robust enough to deal with moments of tension. Differences of view about risk or diagnosis can feel passionately important in the heat of the moment, so we have had to find a way of holding these differences in balance as a recognised part of the dynamics of the group.

The holding function of the group

One aspect of group life that the group members emphasised was the importance of the group as a support over time in the history of our professional lives. Our group is quite unusual in that it has been ongoing for more than 30 years, with some changes in membership, of course, but I imagine other groups offer a similar function. For those of us who are longer term, its bridging function between different episodes in our life has been important in providing continuity. Therapists leave to go on maternity leave or through ill health and return sometime later to refind their place. I felt fortunate to have the group as a secure professional base when my national health service work setting was in turmoil and eventually closed, and I had to make the difficult transition to private practice. Later, others went through similar painful changes, when their services were reorganised or closed, and they were able to draw on memories of my experience and how I got through. So, we see our own struggles reflected in others and learn from how they resolved them.

Difference and commonality

One of the concerns of individual supervision is that the power dynamics of expert and student can undermine a real exchange of ideas and the development of the supervisee. In a well-balanced group, where there is more equality, this is less likely to happen, although the voice of the more experienced may be privileged. If this happens too much, the group becomes unbalanced; each person must feel they have a voice and something to contribute. When I was a newly qualified therapist, a few of us from my year group were able to join an existing group with some more experienced child psychotherapists. I recall how nervous I felt, but how our experience and contributions from our different work settings were welcomed, as they brought a richness to the meetings. With periods away due to life circumstances, I have remained linked to this group ever since. As older members retire new ones join, and the differences in age and experience works well. The 'younger' members bring new insights, energy and enthusiasm and prevent the group becoming stagnant, and the newer recruits feel supported by the experience of us older ones.

Getting the balance between the value of difference and the need for a shared outlook is one of the challenges of a peer group. Peer groups, like friendships, tend to be self-selecting. If the membership is too narrow, the discussion will not truly reflect the diversity of our culture and runs the risk of becoming cut off from the world. Each participant brings knowledge of their own cultural and social realities and life experiences to reflect on the clinical work and this helps us question our assumptions. Yet too much conflict around basic assumptions would make problem-solving together difficult. In our group, there are differences in our ethnicity, our training and our work settings. The majority of the group are employed in national health services but there are a few of us who now only do private work. We are spared the increasing pressures and complexity of public sector employment, but our isolation can be limiting. Similarly, theoretical perspectives could link or divide us, but in practice it is rarely a source of conflict. In the group currently, there are child psychotherapists trained in three differing traditions, Anna Freudian, Kleinian and the Independents, yet when we are discussing clinical cases our theoretical differences do not emerge as an issue for debate. Although we each bring a different viewpoint, there is a sense of cohesion to the group, and the diversity in our background, culture and experience brings a liveliness and breadth to the discussion.

Shared learning

Reviewing my experience of peer group supervision over the years, I realise how I value the process of shared learning, and how important the group has been in my career. When I joined as a newly qualified child therapist, I was looking for the support of colleagues and more experienced members to learn how to manage the clinical work. I now feel more confident in my skill as a psychotherapist, and I supervise and teach many others, but I still value the shared learning process. The 'give and take' involved in supporting each other reduces the sense of inadequacy I can feel in individual supervision, however sympathetic the supervisor, when I am stuck with a case or realise I have overlooked an essential dynamic in the therapeutic relationship. There is always some sense of self-exposure in reading aloud one's work, but alongside this is the excitement of learning something new and the hope one will find a new way forward.

Conclusion

On reflection, it is interesting that when planning this book we knew how important peer-group supervision is to our work, but oddly it was squeezed out of our reckoning until we saw this had happened. Our editorial discussion prompted me to use my experience of peer group supervision for this chapter, and it has been a fascinating process, as previously I had taken it for granted. If I might return to my horticultural metaphor, the pleasure of a mature garden is the pattern that plants create as they grow together over time, their changing structure, shape and colour. The same might be said of a peer group, where the growing relationships between the members allow for conversations to develop, differences to be recognised and individual achievements to become a resource for the group as a whole.

Peer groups over the years have helped me learn how to supervise, as I observe, month by month, differing perspectives and clinical approaches, and how group members sensitively take up issues with each other. The tradition of peer supervision is well grounded in our profession and I expect it will continue to be so for future generations. I hope this chapter will provoke others to share their experiences of peer groups and their ideas about the value they bring to their work.

Acknowledgement

I would like to thank my peer group for their contribution to this chapter and their support and encouragement.

References

Main, T F (1983) The concept of a therapeutic community – variations and vicissitudes. In M Pines (ed.) *The Evolution of Group Analysis* London: Routledge.
Vastardis, M and Phillips, G (2012) On psychoanalytic supervision: avoiding omniscience, encouraging play. In A Horne and M Lanyado (eds.) *Winnicott's Children* London: Routledge.

Chapter 13

A view from the supervisor's chair

Thoughts on turning points and facilitating hope in therapy through face-to-face and online supervision

Monica Lanyado

As a supervisor of clinicians working with severely traumatised children, I have often noticed that there can be a turning point which emerges from times of despair and crisis in the therapeutic process. This chapter is an attempt to explore and draw attention to these transformational moments, which are probably much easier to see from the supervisor's perspective than the therapist's. Becoming more aware of these moments, and trusting them as clinical indicators of change taking place, can help therapists to find their 'bearings' in the midst of what is often a distressing and confusing experience in the consulting room.

With the inevitable strain and awfulness of much of these patients' treatments, alongside our psychoanalytic tendency and need to address the negative and destructive aspects of life, it is often hard for the clinician to recognise the early faint signs of hope and change, particularly when their precursors are shock and despair. But as a supervisor, these transformational moments increasingly stand out for me in the midst of what may otherwise be a chaotic and disturbing session. I now make a point of discussing what may be no more than a clinical hunch of mine at the time – and then waiting as the work proceeds to see whether or not this hunch was justified. In this chapter I am exploring an observational experience within the supervisory process, as opposed to conducting a systematised research project as others have done: in his fascinating paper Carlberg (1997) has used just this type of clinical experience to carefully and retrospectively research turning points in therapy. It is my contention that we need to become much more aware of these transformational moments of hope so that we can facilitate their growth into as much recovery from trauma as is possible. Fromm puts this very clearly:

> To hope is to be ready at every moment for that which is not yet born, and yet not become desperate if there is no birth in our lifetime ... those whose hope is strong see and cherish all signs of life and are ready every moment to help the birth of that which is ready to be born.
>
> (Fromm [1970]2010: 22)

A few pages later, Fromm movingly underlines this statement by writing 'Hope is the psychic concomitant of life and growth' (Fromm [1970]2010: 25).

DOI: 10.4324/9781003297604-16

However, when there has been trauma in a person's life, basic trust in the life force is shattered and, as van der Kolk writes, 'trauma results in a disorder of hope: the capacity of others to provide emotional gratification and security is either undervalued or overvalued' (van der Kolk 1987: 154). In the same volume, Krystal states, 'The trauma victim may suffer from interpersonal numbing a giving up of hope for satisfactory human contact which is the destruction of basic trust' (Krystal 1968, cited in van der Kolk 1987: 154).

It is important to stress that genuine hope is quite different from manic and other defensive forms of hope, and different also from denial. The kind of hope that I am discussing in this chapter follows a time of despair in the therapeutic process. This can also be a time of intimacy and authentic relatedness, when there is an intense sense of the patient and therapist having reached 'rock bottom' in an open and honest way. This is communicated in the therapeutic process itself, and then in the supervisory process which follows the session.

In a broader context, the recovery of hope after trauma is associated with positive emotional growth and positive internal and external change. Hope is the strength of life reasserting itself after a period of bleak 'interpersonal numbing'. We have much to learn about the strength of this 'rhythm of life' from observing the sheer irrepressibility of life after seeming utter devastation; for example, the ability of vegetation to return to the landscape after forest fires, or indeed the first green shoots of spring after the dark and cold of winter.

A view from the supervisor's chair

For many years now, I have been in the interesting and privileged position of offering clinical supervision to psychotherapists working with severely traumatised and neglected children and teenagers. This provides a thought-provoking, intimate and stimulating 'bird's eye view' of many treatments and patient-therapist couples. I have gradually realised that this experience is rather like a 'live/natural' research project, generating observations, ideas and hypotheses within me about the psychoanalytic therapeutic process, which draw on the clinical material that is brought to the supervisory session.

When the supervisory relationship is working well, it plays a significant role in trying to disentangle aspects of the therapist's counter-transference within the safe and protected space of supervision. For example, I have learnt to listen carefully for unusual gaps and holes in the clinical accounts; for times when the supervisee has found it really difficult to write up the notes or has needed extra time to recover from a difficult session. I listen to the emotions expressed by the therapist about the patient and try to encourage the supervisee to examine these feelings within the supervision space, whilst respecting that some of these emotions may be private and need to be examined elsewhere.

Within an established supervisory relationship it becomes possible to think honestly about difficult feelings that the therapist experiences during the session that are on the edge of consciousness and very much the stuff of inchoate emotional communication – both within the patient-therapist relationship and within the therapist-supervisor relationship. When these feelings become alive within the supervision process, this can in turn benefit the patient because what was previously so hard to acknowledge and think about has now been thought about by the therapist together with the supervisor, within the safe and contained confines of supervision. At times such as these, the supervisor helps the therapist to 'hold' difficult and disturbing experiences, and this enables the therapist in turn to hold the difficult and disturbing experiences being expressed by the patient. This combination of experience and reflection within the supervision session can then become part of the conscious awareness of the supervisee when she returns to the clinical situation. Whilst this is helpful to the supervisee, it is also helpful to the supervisor. To draw on the evocative title of Patrick Casement's classic book about 'internal supervision', *On Learning from the Patient*, when I am listening to supervisees' accounts of their work, I am 'learning from the supervisee' (Casement 1985).

Whilst psychoanalytic theory and practice have to address the most destructive aspects of what lies within every one of us, they also rely on the inherent powers of recovery within the individual. Recovery, particularly when potentiated from within the therapeutic relationship, can bring about extraordinary internal transformation. Then the painful and horrific events and relationships that have brought terrible suffering into a traumatised patient's life have not been eradicated, but have been transformed, to varying degrees, into more symbolic forms, enabling a new life narrative to emerge. Unconscious enactments and destructive repetitions of the traumatic events lessen and become more consciously recognised. New emotional development and growth that may have come to a halt following the trauma now become possible.

Michael Parsons captures the essence of this transformative process. He writes:

> Whatever an analyst's orientation, it is the essential *humanity* of the *psychoanalytic* process that helps the human being on the couch to think it might be possible to change. And the specifically *psychoanalytic* quality of the *human* process that the analyst offers is what provides patients with the means to change.
>
> (Parsons 2014: 204, emphasis in original)

In their ground-breaking paper 'Non-interpretive mechanisms in psychoanalytic therapy: the "something more" than interpretation', Stern and his colleagues within the Boston Process of Change Group developed a new language and theory for researching what it is that brings about change in the therapeutic relationship (Stern et al. 1998). This carefully researched paper identifies what the authors term 'moments of meeting' which take place within the 'shared implicit relationship' between the patient and therapist, and they understand these as the 'something more' than interpretation that brings deep change in therapy. I am building on Stern and his colleagues' ideas in what follows, and suggesting that one of the consequences of 'moments of meeting' in therapy and in supervision, is 'moments of hope' that change is possible, even in the aftermath of severe trauma and despair.

As a profession, child and adolescent psychotherapists tend to be caring and thoughtful people even before undertaking the training. Training analysis and supervision build on these personal strengths both during and after training. But we can become worn down, and even burnt out and physically ill because of the demands of the work and the deep ways in which we need to make use of our 'Self' in order to help the patient. We can lose sight of the importance of hope, and indeed of faith in the analytic process itself. We can doubt whether the psychoanalytic process is helpful or suitable for certain cases – and of course at times it may not be.

However perhaps we also risk becoming accommodated to our own strengths, not seeing the positive qualities that we take with us into the consulting room, qualities which I would argue are a significant part of the solid core of us, the 'presence' of the therapist, which our patients perceive as potentially helping them to become less troubled and unhappy (Lanyado 2004). The impact on the therapist who is trying to be as open as possible to so many highly disturbing and distressing communications is profoundly challenging and upsetting, and at times also corrosive. The process of trying to communicate with and to understand such patients can leave the therapist in a pretty desperate state, very much in need of what Sterba (1934) quoted in Casement (1985) calls 'an island of contemplation'. It is these most troubling cases that are often taken to supervision.

Ogden writes that the 'psychoanalytic supervisory relationship is … an indispensable medium through which psychoanalytic knowledge is passed from one generation of psychoanalysts to the next' (Ogden 2009: 31). I want to explore and build on some of Ogden's ideas about supervision, through addressing what happens when the shock waves of traumatic experience come alive within the supervisory process. In addition to the psychoanalytic knowledge that Ogden refers to, emotions that relate to the therapist's counter-transference experience with the patient are re-experienced and begin to be processed during supervision. The counter-transference experience is, in effect, the link between the patient, therapist and supervisor. Again, Ogden has interesting ideas about this, thinking about the process as follows:

> The analyst does not bring the analysand to the supervisory session: rather (with the help of the supervisor) the analyst 'dreams up' the patient in the supervisory session … – 'dreaming up the patient' – in the supervisory setting represents the combined effort of the analyst and the supervisor to bring to life in the supervisions what is true to the analyst's experience of what is occurring at a conscious, preconscious and unconscious level in the analytic relationship.
>
> (Ogden 2009: 34)

This idea of what is co-created within the supervision – 'dreaming up the patient' – is very resonant with Winnicottian theories about how psychotherapy takes place in the transitional space between the therapist and the patient, as a result of their relatedness, and indeed also builds on these concepts. Vastardis and Phillips develop these notions about supervision yet further in their paper about their shared experience of their supervision process, as supervisor and supervisee (Vastardis and Phillips 2012).

With this in mind, 'supervision' almost feels like a misnomer for the process that takes place in the 'supervisory setting'. The *Concise Oxford Dictionary* (1990) describes 'supervision' as to 'superintend, oversee the execution of (a task, etc), or actions or work of a person'. There are very directive, managerial connotations in this definition, which do not sit comfortably with what Ogden is describing as 'dreaming up the patient' or indeed what Winnicott is describing in *Playing and Reality* when thinking about 'where' psychotherapy takes place – that is, the unique, in-between, paradoxical, transitional space of the relationship between patient and therapist, or therapist and supervisor (Winnicott 1971).

Putting together these two sets of ideas about the shock waves of trauma and the supervisory process, where does the notion of 'transforming despair to hope' fit in? Whilst as a supervisor I am in the privileged position of not having to face the tremendously difficult sessions my supervisees are facing daily, it is nevertheless my job to listen with every bit of my being to what they tell me about their work.

Gradually out of the complexity of all that happens within the supervisory session, I have come to feel that a very important part of my function is to notice and to nurture the potential for genuine moments of hope which can, quite paradoxically, emerge from moments of dark despair in the therapeutic process. Not surprisingly, these moments may often not be registered by the therapist, who finds herself in the midst of the very helplessness I am hearing about. As part of the patient-psychotherapist couple, this experience can be very intense at times. I am not talking about empty reassurance from myself to the therapist, but about being alert to the potential for early signs of positive change and hope in the therapeutic process, which can emerge just as things are looking and feeling so dark. These early signs need the therapist's attention and thoughtfulness, but not necessarily the therapist's words through interpretation to the patient. It is a fragile process which has more to do with holding one's breath so as not to disturb it than with trumpeting its arrival.

Of course, the therapist also has to be alert to negative change in the patient, particularly with severely traumatised patients, and to be aware of the undertow of the unconscious pressure to repeat traumatic experiences in the present. It would be foolish to seem to assert that all despair can ultimately lead to hope. Sadly, some terrible situations do go from bad to worse, and as therapists we have to face these situations in which psychotherapy cannot be of help to the child or family realistically.

In particular, as the example later in this chapter demonstrates, when there has been extreme trauma, and the therapist describes a shocking experience in the therapy session, the shock wave of the trauma may be experienced in a particular way by the supervisor through a 'moment of meeting' within the supervision session, when discussing the clinical material. Just like a tsunami that sweeps over the landscape leaving terrible destruction, the shock waves of trauma can decimate the ability to think, and the therapist can briefly experience a sense of disintegration and collapse of all boundaries, which puts her in deep contact with the experience of the traumatised patient. These experiences often need to be discussed in supervision, but this can be a revealing, emotional and intense experience within the supervisory relationship itself. When this happens, it can feel as if the therapist/supervisor is 'pierced' by the projections, in a way that confirms that what is being communicated has been deeply understood and felt by the other (Horne 2009; Heimann 1950). The powerful authenticity of what I have come to think of as 'moments of meeting' within the supervisory relationship can help to deepen the whole quality of that relationship. They are moments of change and of hope in the supervisory relationship and, as I illustrate later in this chapter, they can lead to turning points and transformational moments in the patient-therapist relationship.

Shock waves and defences

The traumatised child's vulnerability, pain and helplessness are dreadful and it can take quite a while before the full extent of this really gets through to the therapist. When it does, deeply distressing feelings are stirred in the therapist which need to be explored within the supervisory process. It is precisely because external reality, both past and present, is so complex that it must be carefully thought about and absorbed by the therapist if the child's distress and predicament are to be fully understood. It is also why, in my view, case 'management' concerning these complex external realities must be discussed within supervision, alongside concentrated psychoanalytic listening to the child's communications from the internal world, communications that may, of course, take many forms. The epicentre of the shock wave is in the child patient. The adults and other children in the child's world are made very aware of this by the child's distressed, disturbing and violent behaviour. Parents, foster and adoptive parents, residential care staff, teachers, doctors, siblings, foster siblings and classmates all experience these shock waves in some form – for example, as verbal and physical aggression, distressing and distressed communications, manic and highly reactive behaviour.

The therapist experiences the shock waves in a different way and is trained to try to listen psychoanalytically and to receive with body and soul all that is being communicated. In everyday life and relationships with others, despite the best will in the world, the behaviour and emotional communication coming from the child may simply become unmanageable and, as a result, people may need to defend themselves from what is projected into them by the child. Then there is no possibility of the child's communication being fully received, let alone processed in any way by another human being. The child remains shut out and isolated from 'satisfactory human contact' (as in the above quote from Krystal 1968: 154). And, even though it is the therapist's job to receive the communications as fully as she can, there are often times when it is all too much for the therapist as well. During training, and at other times in the therapist's professional life, it will be possible for her to take these overwhelming experiences to their own analyst to express, explore and digest. But much of the time these difficulties will be taken to supervision or colleagues in the clinic team. If this does not happen, there is a risk of the therapist becoming less and less open to the child's communications of trauma and more and more defended against them. These are the times when hope can shut down. It is part of the supervisor's work to try to fully experience the impact of the shock wave as communicated by the supervisee, and then to stand back and try to think about the experience. This can help the supervisee to remain as open as possible to what is being communicated by the patient; more receptive, less defended and more contained as a result of supervision, particularly at a time of crisis.

Frances Tustin, writing about her work with children in autistic states of mind, also reminds us of the importance of maintaining hope. She writes 'As I see it, in everything that we do, we need to come down on the side of life and hope' (Tustin 1986: 294). In the following examples from supervision, only a very brief case history will be given, and facts that do not affect the essence of the case material have been altered in order to protect the patient's and the supervisee's confidentiality. The supervisees and their colleagues involved with the patient have given their permission for this supervision to be used to demonstrate the processes I am focusing on in this chapter for which I am very grateful. By focusing on the processes I hope that it is possible to avoid getting too involved in the case material itself and instead focus on what is happening in the supervisory relationship.

Brief history

Tina was born to a mother who had diagnosed mental health problems. There were a number of foster placements as mother was often unable to look after Tina. Eventually a kinship carer was identified but unfortunately after a few months it emerged that a close friend of his who had regular contact with Tina had been charged with a sexual offence against children. It was possible that this person had abused Tina but this was never proven, however Tina did at times behave in very sexualised and boundaryless ways. When Tina was four she was adopted. She started psychotherapy when she was six and a half because her violent outbursts were often unmanageable and unfathomable to her adoptive parents. Her adoptive parents were seen regularly at the clinic, and there were regular reviews with the psychotherapist.

Clinical extract

The clinical extract below is from when Tina had been in therapy for about a year. There had been very little overtly sexualised clinical material until a few weeks before this session, and the transference relationship was conflicted but could include brief and valuable times of intimacy. This suggested that the 'core complex' of longing for and dreading intimacy that Glasser describes, was beginning to soften (Glasser 1998). Tina was still very traumatised and various small triggers could cause panics when she would try to hide in the room, clearly in terror. She could also suddenly attack her therapist in shocking ways and had scratched her, broken her glasses and tried to strangle her. Despite this there was a real fondness and good communication between them as well as a gradual growing capacity for intimacy.

The following material came after a few sessions in which the therapist started to wonder to herself whether Tina could be beginning to try to share her conscious memories of being sexually abused. This became explicit in a shocking way in this session. The following clinical excerpt comes roughly halfway through the session and came after Tina had already tried to approach the memories of sexual abuse several times through her play, but had run out of the room or diverted to other play because, in her words, she 'needed a break'. The play she was finding it so hard to keep going with, was about some little 'piggies' who were in a bath. I quote from the therapist's session notes:

> She goes back to the piggies. I wonder if she can show me what happens next. They are in the bath and the tiger cub comes in. I comment that there is a lot I am not sure about but I wonder if something is happening to the piggies. She goes to the couch and lies down facing me. She pulls up her skirt around her waist and bending her knees lets them fall open so that her knickers are exposed. She fingers these and looks at me. I feel shocked. I say that I think she is showing me something about the piggies and their knickers and their private area. Perhaps someone did something to them that they didn't like. I am speaking very gently but feel as if the next part of the session is a bit of a blur.

Supervision session

The supervisory relationship was well established and we had often wondered when more explicit sexual material would emerge in a session. So it was not as if the therapist was unprepared for what happened in the session. However, it was nevertheless deeply shocking and upsetting for the therapist who not only found the rest of the session to be a 'bit of a blur', but was clearly upset during our supervision about the impact this material had on her. She had found it very hard to put the patient out of her mind in the time between the session and the supervision. The 'shock wave' had really got through to her and rolled on into our supervisory session.

I am very grateful to this supervisee for our discussions whilst I was preparing this chapter. We talked about what happened during this supervision (for which we both had our supervision notes), as one that had stood out in my mind and in hers, as a powerful experience and what could be described as a 'moment of meeting' in supervision. The supervisee felt that the supervision helped her to be in touch with her own feelings of terrible helplessness as she listened to and watched her patient. The supervision helped us to relate this to the child's terrible feelings of helplessness at the time of the suspected abuse, as well as her utter aloneness. Possibly when the child became able to share her experience so rawly with her therapist, and with such an impact, the communication was received fully and forcefully by her therapist, and so was communicated powerfully in turn during the supervision. This is the 'piercing' experience to which Horne refers (personal communication 2015).[1] I also find Ogden's idea of 'dreaming up the patient' very helpful here (Ogden 2009). Tina seemed vividly present in the supervision room at the time as we talked about the session.

I had the advantage of being at one step removed from the shocking experience that the supervisee bought to supervision, and was able to think about what had happened, as well as to draw on my experience of similar cases. But essentially the work of fully understanding and appreciating the child's traumatic emotional state was appreciated within our supervisory relationship, through the moment of meeting that was experienced between the supervisee and myself. What then rolled on from the supervision into the treatment was co-created by the two of us, and then the two of them – therapist and patient.

During the supervision itself, we were also able to note the supervisee's defences coming to the fore. She had a sense of being 'in a blur' possibly connecting to a mild dissociative state which blurred the impact of the sexual abuse that was revealed through the play. The shock that she felt through witnessing this play seemed to confirm the significance of what her patient was communicating without words. The 'blur' possibly also gave some indication of the defences the child might have used at the time of the traumatic experience, which may very well have included dissociation. We were able to think about the value of these defences at the time of the trauma taking place – but also the need for these defences to soften so that less extreme defences could gradually come into play, over time. This applied both to the patient and to the therapist in her efforts to really listen to and receive what the patient was communicating.

Searles (quoted in Ogden (2009: 35)) refers to this process:

> The (conscious and unconscious) processes at work currently in the *relationship between* patient and therapist are often reflected in the (conscious and unconscious) *relationship between* therapist and supervisor …
>
> (Searles 1955: 159, emphasis in original)

Ogden also refers to this process, describing the connection between the analytic process and the supervisory process as being like two facets of a single set of conscious and unconscious relationships, internal and external, involving the supervisor, supervisee and patient (Ogden 2009).

Importantly, as if to confirm the significance of the communications between patient, therapist and supervisor around this experience in the consulting room, the supervisions that followed this one indicated that Tina was increasingly able to trust her therapist and to dare to get closer to her. There was a new feeling of hope in the treatment for the therapist and child, as well as for her adoptive parents and within the supervisory process.

Online supervision: despair and hope

Over many years when physical distance made face-to-face supervision impossible, some psychotherapists have found phone supervision to be helpful. This way of working was felt to be 'good-enough' for many long-lasting supervisory relationships. These psychotherapists learnt how to make the most of their ability to listen particularly carefully to each other, whilst not having the facial and bodily cues of the face-to-face relationship. Intonation, silences, gaps in accounts of sessions as well as the personal aspect of the supervisory relationship could be understood as being of significance by the supervisor.

The Covid pandemic which launched so many of us into the world of online psychotherapy and supervision resulted in additional visual cues which built on the auditory phone supervision experience. As we are unlikely ever to return fully to our previous face-to-face work, it is helpful in the context of this chapter to think about how well supervision works online. During the pandemic, it was noticeable that flexibility of many previously very firm boundaries around psychotherapybecame helpful and indeed necessary if therapy was to be at all viable. But can the flexibility or elasticity of such a boundary stretch too far so that it snaps and therapy is no longer viable as it is no longer held sufficiently, as suggested by Ryz and Wilson (1999)? These questions are explored in the following example. I am again grateful to my colleagues for their permission to include our work in this chapter.

Brief history

The ten-year-old female patient was referred during the Covid lockdown because of severe traumatic experiences, the repercussions of which were rapidly becoming impossible for her loving family to cope with. Because of the seriousness of her problems she was seen face to face at the clinic. This intelligent and thoughtful girl knew she needed therapy despite her ambivalence about it, and her parents were prepared to go to considerable lengths to bring her to the clinic three times weekly. During lockdown the family situation could become so stressful that at times when the girl's intense distress and rage became totally unmanageable, she would be sent from her family home to the home of extended family at little or no notice. However, this extended family, who were able to and wanted to help, lived in another part of the country, a long way from the clinic. When the patient went to live with the extended family during lockdown, the therapist tried to continue with the three times weekly online work, but this became increasingly devoid of meaning until the therapist eventually felt that her patient's sudden external temporary moving home made therapy non-viable. The supervision sessions also took place almost exclusively online because of physical distance and Covid restrictions.

Supervision session

There had been yet another very sudden move of the patient to her distant extended family since our last supervision session and the therapist felt distressed about the impact of what was bound to be experienced by the patient as a result of yet another rejection by her family. The therapist felt it was no longer right to offer therapy in these unstable circumstances. This was during a period when face-to-face work in the clinic had become possible again but was painfully disrupted each time the girl was suddenly transported to her distant extended family – where she nevertheless felt more contained than in her family home. Whilst the therapist was very committed to the work, she felt it was wrong to continue to offer intensive therapy in these circumstances and very reluctantly felt she had to discuss this with the parents. In the supervision we discussed other psychotherapy treatment plans as well as the need to work out how to bring the three times weekly work to an end. The therapist was very despairing and disappointed that this needed to happen, but nevertheless convinced that the three times weekly work could not continue in its current form, against the backdrop of such instability in the patient's external world.

In our discussions, whilst recognising the need to set up an urgent meeting with the parents together with the parent worker, we thought that if at all possible, prior to this meeting it would be helpful if the supervisee, her co-worker who worked with the parents and myself were able to meet online to think through what was the wisest path forward. To my surprise it seemed that the family had concurrently reached a similar conclusion about the girl's living arrangements so that her life was less chaotic and had some regularity in it. The hastily arranged meeting with the parents, which happened before the therapist, her co-worker and I met, ensured that the girl would reliably be able to have her face-to-face sessions again whilst spending weekends and holidays with her extended family. The work with the parent worker continued to support the family.

It is important to note that during the supervision, due to the supervisee's powerful and courageous communication of despair, I had also felt despair about the intensive psychotherapeutic work continuing. As an essentially hopeful supervisor, this was unusual. With hindsight, perhaps the honesty with which the supervisee was able to share her feelings about the work with me was a moment of meeting in the supervision which in turn enabled her to be frank with the parents about their daughter's living arrangements and her ongoing therapy. Space does not permit me to enlarge on thoughts about the synchronicity of the parents' change in plans and the therapist's. But suffice it to say, the therapy has since moved forward again and the underlying trauma is once more coming to the surface of the clinical material. Pragmatically, the new living arrangements and the therapy are working, for now.

During the pandemic our professional body worked hard to help all of us to keep thinking and discussing the impact of Covid and working online on our work. As a supervisor, I have felt supported and held by the thoughtfulness of what has been offered. This has greatly helped me to find ways of thinking about the complex issues involved in this example.

Conclusion

Perhaps the moment of hope arises when someone who desperately needs help dares to cry out to someone who is prepared to listen. In this respect, a crisis may contain the seeds of a turning point for the better. Both of the above patients managed to communicate their trauma powerfully to their therapists, who in turn communicated this to me through 'dreaming up the patient' in their supervisions. In my 'view from the supervisor's chair', this was possible in online supervision, as well as in face-to-face supervision.

Note: This chapter is an adaptation of an earlier paper (Lanyado 2016), and book chapter (Lanyado 2018), adding thoughts and an example from online supervision.

Note

1 Conversation with Anne Horne, 15 May 2015

References

Carlberg, G (1997) Laughter opens the door: turning points in child psychotherapy. *Journal of Child Psychotherapy 23 (3)*: 331–349.
Casement, P (1985) *On Learning from the Patient* London and New York: Tavistock Publications.
Concise Oxford Dictionary (1990) Oxford: Clarendon Press.
Fromm, E ([1968]2010) *The Revolution of Hope: Toward a Humanised Technology* New York: Harper & Row and American Mental Health Foundation.
Glasser, M (1998) On violence: a preliminary communication. *International Journal of Psycho-Analysis 79 (5)*: 887–902.
Heimann, P (1950) On counter-transference. *International Journal of Psycho-Analysis 31*:81–84.
Horne, A (2009) From intimacy to acting out: assessment and consultation about a dangerous child. In A Horne and M Lanyado (eds.) *Through Assessment to Consultation* London and New York: Routledge.
Krystal, H (1968) *Massive Psychic Trauma* New York: International Universities Press.
Lanyado, M (2004) *The Presence of the Therapist: Treating Childhood Trauma* Hove and New York: Brunner-Routledge.
Lanyado, M (2016) Transforming despair to hope in the treatment of extreme trauma: a view from the supervisor's chair. *Journal of Child Psychotherapy 42 (2)*: 107–121.
Lanyado, M (2018) Transforming despair to hope in the treatment of extreme trauma: a view from the supervisor's chair. In M Lanyado *Transforming Despair to Hope: Reflections on the Psychotherapeutic Process with Severely Neglected and Traumatised Children* London and New York: Routledge.

Ogden, T (2009) On psychoanalytic supervision. In *Rediscovering Psychoanalysis: Thinking and Dreaming, Learning and Forgetting*. New Library of Psychoanalysis Series. London and New York: Routledge.

Parsons, Michael (2014) An Independent theory of technique. In *Living Psychoanalysis: From Theory to Experience* Hove and New York: Routledge.

Ryz, P and Wilson, J (1999) Endings as gain: the capacity to end and its role in creating space for growth. *Journal of Child Psychotherapy 25*: 379–403.

Searles, H (1955) The informational value of the supervisor's emotional experiences. In *Collected Papers on Schizophrenia and Related Subjects* New York: International Universities Press.

Sterba, R (1934) The fate of the ego in analytic therapy. *International Journal of Psycho-Analysis 15*: 117–126.

Stern, D, Sander, L, Nahum, J, Harrison, A, Lyons-Ruth, K, Morgan, A, Bruschweiler-Stern, N and Tronich, E (1998) Non-interpretive mechanisms in psychoanalytic therapy: the 'something more' than interpretation. *International Journal of Psycho-Analysis 79*: 903–921.

Tustin, F (1986) *Autistic Barriers in Neurotic Patients* London: Karnac.

van der Kolk, B A (1987) *Psychological Trauma* Washington: American Psychiatric Press.

Vastardis, M and Phillips, G (2012) On psychoanalytic supervision: avoiding omniscience, encouraging play. In A Horne and M Lanyado (eds.) *Winnicott's Children* Hove: Routledge.

Winnicott, D W (1965) *The Maturational Processes and the Facilitating Environment* London: Hogarth Press and Institute of Psycho-Analysis.

Winnicott, D W (1971) *Playing and Reality* London: Penguin Books.

Index

For Product Safety Concerns and Information please contact our EU
representative GPSR@taylorandfrancis.com
Taylor & Francis Verlag GmbH, Kaufingerstraße 24, 80331 München, Germany

www.ingramcontent.com/pod-product-compliance
Lightning Source LLC
Chambersburg PA
CBHW052007270326
41929CB00015B/2824

9 781032 286006